Clinical
Pharmacokinetics:
The MCQ
Approach

Clinical Pharmacokinetics: The MCQ Approach

STEPHEN H. CURRY, Ph.D.

College of Pharmacy
University of Florida
Gainesville
Florida

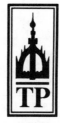

THE TELFORD PRESS
Caldwell, New Jersey

THE TELFORD PRESS, INC.
285 Bloomfield Avenue, Caldwell, New Jersey, 07006

Library of Congress Cataloging-in-Publication Data

Curry, Stephen H.
   Clinical pharmacokinetics.

   Bibliography: p.
   1. Pharmacokinetics—Problems, exercises, etc.
2. Pharmacokinetics—Examinations, questions, etc.
I. Title. [DNLM: 1. Chemistry, Pharmaceutical—
problems. 2. Drugs—metabolism—problems. 3. Kinetics—
problems. 4. Pharmacology, Clinical—problems.
QV 18 C9767c]
RM301.5.C86 1987   615'.7'076   87-19435
ISBN 0-936923-03-2
ISBN 0-936923-02-4 (pbk.)

Contents

Preface

Pharmacokinetics adopts the modifier "clinical" when it becomes concerned with the analysis of drug disposition data obtained from human subjects, both healthy volunteers and patients, and when the results of such analyses are applied in patient care programs. The accumulation of skills relevant to such work is not easy. Constant practice with problem solving exercises, akin to that required in learning a foreign language, is necessary.

This book is a compilation of practice problems, all in the field of clinical pharmacokinetics. Its objectives are: (i) to provide students with an opportunity to work revision problems with special emphasis on understanding how errors are made and (ii) to provide teachers with guidance on the use of multiple-choice questions as both a teaching/learning medium and a testing mechanism. The emphasis on teaching and learning is important and intended. Working problems is an excellent method of developing skills in clinical pharmacokinetics.

The multiple-choice question (MCQ) style is used throughout the book. This is partly to demonstrate the fact that MCQ-style testing is possible in this field of biomedical science. However, there is an additional advantage. MCQ-style questions can be designed to focus attention on plausible but incorrect answers. This presentation of the correct answer among distractors can be used to demonstrate how common errors are made, such as by using wrong units, failing to change time from hours to minutes when needed, etc. A valuable learning experience results from a student calculating a wrong answer and then discovering why he or she obtained this incorrect answer. MCQ problems are as relevant to reasoning exercises as they are to factual recall.

This particular book has MCQ problems of four types. Part I presents the reader with data for graphing. Properties of the system generating the data are sought, and the correct answer can, generally speaking, only be derived after the data are drawn on graph paper. Part II presents the reader with single-answer calculation questions. Questions in Parts I and II can be completed satisfactorily using the equations in the Introduction.

The first eight problems in Part II are concerned with the very few arithmetical/calculator techniques required for success in clinical pharmacokinetics. The basic needs are:

(i) The ability to handle logarithms and exponentials, including

i

clearly understanding the difference between *common* and *natural* logarithms; and

(ii) the ability to use a linear regression program in a scientific calculator.

Additionally, it is useful if the practitioner of clinical pharmacokinetics can write a simple simulation or analysis program for an inexpensive programmable pocket calculator.

Part III comprises single-answer factual questions. Confirmation of the validity of the answers given will require reading of at least one, perhaps several, of the references listed in the Appendix. Parts IV and V are made up of multiple-answer factual questions, in which any number of answer statements (1–4) is correct in each question and with which a "decoding" system is used to generate a single-letter answer for the question as a whole. All four styles of question are useful in both learning and testing, although the questions of the type in Part III are open to criticism for presenting the reader with 80% false information. I have deliberately avoided use of five-answer questions in which any number of answers is correct, as such questions are little more than multi-part true/false questions.

In preparation for the study of Part V, it will be necessary for the reader to examine the literature concerned with the effect of various physiological and pathological factors on pharmacokinetic observations. For each question in Part V, one or more references to recent papers are given as a literature entry point. To be satisfied that the answer given is correct, the reader may need to "read around" the entry point paper, either by pursuing references in that paper or by conducting a formal search. The reader will probably need also to consult the references in the Appendix. There is no attempt to be comprehensive in this section, which is designed primarily to illustrate an available style of problem setting.

The mathematical questions relate to some 50 core equations. These equations are set out in the introductory section. Most of the simple problems met in the practice of clinical pharmacokinetics can be solved using these equations. Users of this book should develop a working knowledge of this initial section and then refine this knowledge as they work the problems. Once mastery of the introductory section and the problems is achieved, graduation to a higher level of personal study of pharmacokinetics will not prove difficult. No particular sequence of use of the sections of this book is needed, except that Part I should be studied first, as it is designed to focus attention on the pictorial aspect of pharmacokinetics, in that the commonly observed graph shapes are all presented. Even when a problem is presented only in sentences, it is advisable before seeking a solution to develop at least a mental picture of the system described. This is illustrated with special emphasis in problem 58.

The MCQ problems in this book deal with the relevant mathematical models, the physiological and biochemical basis for clinical pharmacokinetics, and the biological and pathological factors which influence the intensity and duration of drug action. As an appendix, I have listed some 30 core reference books, key papers, etc., both to aid in the use of this book and as the basis for reading at a higher level when this book has served its purpose. This book is *not* a complete text in clinical pharmacokinetics—most readers will need to consult one or more of the standard textbooks at the same time as working the problems in this book. Also, Part V is deliberately designed to force its readers into their libraries.

Most of the problems in this book have been used in exercises of various types by approximately 12 separate groups of advanced professional and postgraduate students at the University of Florida, during the period 1980–1987. I am grateful to my students for their help, sometimes unwitting, in developing these problems. Also, some of the problems undoubtedly reflect input from professional colleagues, to whom I am especially grateful and from whom I beg forgiveness if one or more of their contributions has inadvertently emerged as if it were my own invention. Finally, I wish to thank Judy Hulton for her patience and skill during the typing of the text of this book.

Gainesville, Florida   Stephen H. Curry, Ph.D.
Autumn, 1987.

INTRODUCTION

Fundamental Pharmacokinetic Equations

Pharmacokinetics starts with two concepts, the half-life and the apparent volume of distribution.

The *half-life* $(T_{1/2})$ is the time taken for the drug concentration to decline by 50%. In the simplest cases, the half-life is the same regardless of dose. It is rarely an absolute constant, being affected by physiological, pathological, and environmental factors, so that individual patients have their own half-life values for each drug. Note that:

90% of the body content is lost in $3.32 \times T_{1/2}$
95% of the body content is lost in $4.32 \times T_{1/2}$
99% of the body content is lost in $6.65 \times T_{1/2}$

These figures are often rounded up to 4, 5 and 7, with the statement that: "X% is lost *within* $n \times T_{1/2}$."

The *apparent volume of distribution* (Vd) is the volume of fluid which the drug would occupy if it was evenly distributed through that volume at the concentration measured in plasma. Thus it is possible for Vd to be a recognizable volume, such as plasma volume (0.05 l/kg), extracellular fluid (0.2 l/kg), or total body water (0.7 l/kg). However, it is commonly an unreal volume, such as one intermediate between two of the examples above. Vd can even exceed total body volume, hence the use of the adjective "apparent." This results when there is preferential binding to tissues at the expense of plasma.

Fundamental Pharmacokinetic Equations

First-order case

This is the case in which the decay of drug concentration is mono-exponential, and for which

$$Cp_t = Cp_0 e^{-k_{el}t}$$

in which Cp_t is concentration at time t, Cp_0 is concentration at time zero (a theoretical concentration, obtained by back-extrapolating concentration/time data to the y-intercept), k_{el} is the rate constant of decline of concentration, and t is the time. It should be noted that

$$\ln Cp_t = \ln Cp_0 - k_{el}t$$

This equation describes a straight-line graph from which k_{el} is obtained by linear regression or by calculation of the slope using standard techniques. The half-life is given by the equation

$$T_{1/2} = 0.693 / k_{el}$$

and the apparent volume of distribution is given by the equation

$$Vd = Dose / Cp_0$$

Note that this gives a Vd with volume units. If the dose is measured in weight/weight units (e.g., mg/kg), the units of Vd are volume/weight (e.g., l/kg).

The total body clearance (Cl) is given by the following equation:

$$Cl = Vd \cdot k_{el}$$

Note that clearance as defined here is the clearance of the drug from its apparent volume of distribution by all processes. It is sometimes termed systemic clearance, and may be given the symbol Cl_s (where s stands for systemic). It is also sometimes termed "total body clearance" and given the symbol Cl_{TOT} or Cl_{tot} where TOT or tot indicates "total." The use of the word "total" refers to Cl_s being the sum of all clearances (see later).

It is useful to measure the area under a curve (graph) of concentration in plasma against time. The symbols for area under the curve are AUC and area. For intravenous doses

$$AUC = Cp_0 / k_{el} = Dose / Vd \cdot k_{el} = Dose / Cl$$

Hence, Cl = Dose/Area. AUC for oral doses can be computed by integration or by using the trapezoidal rule. For oral doses, "Dose" must be corrected to allow for incomplete absorption.

For oral doses, the following holds true:

$$Cp_t = \frac{F \cdot D}{Vd} \cdot \frac{k_a}{k_a - k_{el}} [e^{-k_{el}t} - e^{-k_a t}]$$

in which F is the fraction of the dose reaching the general circulation, sometimes called "bioavailability," D is the dose, and k_a is the rate constant of first-order absorption. The time of the maximum concentration (t_{max}) is given by the equation

$$t_{max} = \frac{1}{k_a - k_{el}} \ln \frac{k_a}{k_{el}}$$

The concentration at t_{max} (C_{max}) is obtainable by substituting t_{max} into the equation for Cp for the oral dose. In that equation, $FD/Vd = Cp_0$, in which Cp_0 is the theoretical concentration obtained by back-extrapolation of the decay phase of the oral dose growth and decay curve to the y-axis. Also, k_a often exceeds k_{el} by a large amount, and the following is commonly seen:

$$Cp_t = Cp_0[e^{-k_{el}t} - e^{-k_a t}]$$

It should be noted that the Cp_0 in this equation can, but rarely will, be the same as Cp_0 following an intravenous dose of the same magnitude as the oral dose.

Zero-order Decay

Occasionally, drug concentrations will be seen to decline at a constant rate. In such a case, after an intravenous dose or after an oral dose when the growth phase is disregarded,

$$Cp_t = Cp_0 + (-Rt)$$

in which R is the constant rate of decay.

Zero-Order Infusions (with First-Order Decay)

In this case the drug concentration increases at an ever decreasing rate until a plateau concentration is reached. At the time of the plateau, input (dosing) is in balance with output (elimination) and the body is said to be in a steady state with respect to the drug. The plateau concentration, the steady-state concentration (Cp_{ss}), is given by the equation

$$Cp_{ss} = k_0/Vd \cdot k_{el}$$

in which k_0 is the input rate. Note that during the phase of increase in Cp at an ever decreasing rate:

90% of steady state is reached after $3.32 \times T_{1/2}$
95% of steady state is reached after $4.32 \times T_{1/2}$
99% of steady state is reached after $6.65 \times T_{1/2}$

These figures are often rounded up to 4, 5, and 7.

Prior to the achievement of steady state, the following holds true:

$$Cp_t = k_0/Vd \cdot k_{el}[1 - e^{-k_{el}t}]$$

and at steady state, the following is true:

$$k_0 = Cl \cdot Cp_{ss}$$

Steady State (Oral Cases)

The equations for intravenous doses apply, except that Cp_{ss} is the mean of a fluctuating pattern with peaks and troughs consequent on the pulsed nature of oral dosing. Also, the input rate (k_0) is now a daily (for example) dosing rate.

The area under the curve at steady state (AUC_{ss}) is given by:

$$AUC_{ss} = Cp_{ss} \cdot \tau$$

where AUC_{ss} is the area under the curve for a single dosage interval and τ is the dosing interval. AUC_{ss} is equal to $AUC_{(0 \rightarrow \infty)}$ measured after a single dose; $AUC_{(0 \rightarrow \infty)}$ is the area from zero time (time of dosing) to the time when the concentration is zero. This is computed using the trapezoidal rule. Fluctuation at steady state is given by

$$\text{Fluctuation } (\%) = \frac{\text{Peak concentration} - \text{Trough concentration}}{\text{Peak concentration}} \times 100$$

However, some investigators prefer to use a different definition,

$$\text{Fluctuation } (\%) = \frac{\text{Peak}}{\text{Trough}} \times 100$$

which results in a different value. In multiple dosing at steady state, when $\tau = T_{1/2}$, concentration will double after each dose and fall by 50% from peak to trough. If $\tau > T_{1/2}$, there will be more fluctuation; if $\tau < T_{1/2}$, there will be less.

Concentrations following initial doses and those at steady state are related as follows:

$$Cp_{ss} = Cp_{\text{First dose}}/f$$

where Cp_{ss} and $Cp_{\text{First dose}}$ are measured during the respective dosage intervals at the same time (i.e., both peak, both trough, or both means), and f is fractional fall from peak to trough [(peak − trough)/peak].

Organ Uptake

Considering the case of an organ removing part of the drug from the blood passing through it,

$$\text{Uptake} = Q\left[\frac{Ca - Cv}{Ca}\right]$$

where Q is blood flow to the organ, Ca is the drug concentration in the arterial supply to the organ, and Cv is the drug concentration in the venous drainage of the organ.

Clearance (generally applied only to eliminating organs) can be defined in the same way. Thus clearance and uptake both have units of volume/time (volume of blood from which the drug is completely removed in unit time). Thus clearances in pharmacokinetics can be calculated if arterial and venous drug concentration data are available. This, of course, is rare. Clearances are usually obtained from venous plasma drug concentration decay (see earlier) and from measurements of drug concentrations in excreta (see next section).

Renal Clearance

The use of the term clearance in relation to the kidney predates use of the term in relation to plasma level decay. Renal clearance (Cl_R) is given by the equation

$$Cl_R = \frac{\text{Concentration of drug in urine} \times \text{Urine flow rate}}{\substack{\text{Concentration of drug in plasma at midpoint} \\ \text{of urine collection time}}}$$

$$= \frac{UV}{P}$$

Clearances and rate constants (but not half-life values) are additive, so that, for a drug eliminated partly in urine and partly by metabolism in the liver, the following applies:

$$Cl_{TOT} = Cl_R + Cl_H$$

where Cl_H is "hepatic clearance." Also,

$$k_{el} = k_R + k_M$$

where k_R and k_M are first-order rate constants of renal and hepatic elimination. The consequence of this is that if Cl_R is measured directly and Cl_{TOT} is measured from the half-life of decay of concentration in plasma, an evaluation can be made of Cl_H, the clearance in an essentially inaccessible organ.

Hepatic Extraction Ratio (E)

This is given by the equation

$$E = Cl_i/(Q_H + Cl_i)$$

where Q_H is hepatic blood flow and Cl_i is the intrinsic clearance of the drug in question in the absence of blood flow limitations. Note that

$$Cl_H = Q_H E$$

so that

$$Cl_H = Q_H\left[\frac{Cl_i}{Q_H + Cl_i}\right]$$

and that Cl_i is greater than Cl_H. Note also:

$$Cl_i = \alpha Cl_i'$$

where α is the free (nonbound) fraction in plasma and Cl_i' is the intrinsic clearance in the absence of protein binding (or, for that matter, blood flow) restrictions. Thus

$$Cl_i' > Cl_i > Cl_H$$

When Cl_i is high, E is high and

$$Cl_H = Q_H$$

When Cl_i is low, E is low and

$$Cl_H = Cl_i$$

Michaelis–Menten Cases

Drug elimination sometimes follows Michaelis–Menten kinetics:

$$\text{Rate of elimination} = \frac{V_{max} \cdot S}{K_m + S}$$

where V_{max} is the maximum possible rate of change occurring at very high substrate concentrations (actually zero order), S is the substrate concentration, and K_m is the substrate concentration at half-maximum velocity. There is no useful integrated form of this equation describing a concentration/time graph.

If a patient is dosed to steady state with a drug showing Michaelis–Menten kinetics, at steady state

$$k_0 = V_{max} - \left[\frac{k_0}{Cp_{ss}} \cdot K_m \right]$$

Thus, in this case, Cp_{ss} and time to steady state are dependent on k_0, K_m, and V_{max} (and also on Vd). Clearance is not a constant, nor is time to steady state. However, if different dosing rates are used, each inducing a different Cp_{ss}, then a graph of k_0 against k_0/Cp_{ss} is a straight line of slope $-K_m$ and intercept V_{max}. The time to reach 90% of steady state ($T_{90\%}$) is given by:

$$T_{90\%} = \frac{K_m \cdot Vd}{(V_{max} - k_0)^2} (2.303 \, V_{max} - 0.9 \, k_0)$$

Two-compartment cases

The equation for double exponential decline of the drug concentration in plasma is

$$Cp_t = Ae^{-\alpha t} + Be^{-\beta t}$$

where α and β are the rate constants of the initial (faster) and later (slower) exponential phases of plasma level decay and A and B are intercepts of the two construction lines used in determining α and β.

Loading doses

It is sometimes desirable to immediately induce the steady-state concentration that would normally have been obtained once 4–7 ×

$T_{1/2}$ had elapsed. This is achieved by using volume of distribution data for intravenous dosing:

$$\text{Loading dose} = Cp_{ss} \times Vd$$

For oral dosing:

$$\text{Loading dose} = Cp_{ss} \times Vd \times \frac{1}{F}$$

When the half-life is equal to the oral dosing interval ($T_{1/2} = \tau$), the loading dose is twice the planned maintenance dose. A figure of 1.44 times the maintenance doses is commonly discussed in this context. This follows from:

$$Cp_{ss} = \frac{k_0}{Vd \cdot k_{el}} = \frac{FD}{Cl \cdot \tau}$$

$$k_0 = FD/\tau$$

$$Vd \cdot k_{el} = \frac{Vd \times 0.693}{T_{1/2}}$$

$$Cp_{ss} = \frac{F \cdot D \cdot T_{1/2}}{\tau \times Vd \times 0.693} = \frac{FD}{Vd \times 0.693}$$

$$\text{Loading dose} = Cp_{ss} \cdot Vd$$

$$1/0.693 = 1.44$$

$$\text{Loading Dose} = FD \times 1.44$$

$$Cp_{ss} = \frac{FD}{Vd \cdot k_{el} \cdot \tau}$$

Note that D here is the maintenance dose and that Cp_{ss} is the mean plasma concentration at steady state.

Use of the 1.44 figure gives a concentration somewhat below the desired steady-state concentration. It leads to induction of a pre-maintenance dose concentration equal to the mean steady-state concentration. Strictly, therefore, the first maintenance dose should follow the loading dose at an interval of approximately $0.5 \times \tau$. Alternatively, the loading dose should be twice the maintenance dose.

Kinetics of Drug Effects

Assuming that the central portion of a graph relating response and log dose is linear, intensity of effect (I) is given by

$$I = a + b \log Qd$$

where Qd is dose and a and b are constants. Combining this equation with the standard equation for the decay of plasma concentration of drug gives

$$I_t = I_0 - \frac{k_{el}bt}{2.303}$$

where I_t is intensity at time t and I_0 is intensity at time zero, immediately after an intravenous dose has equilibrated within the body, and t is time since time zero. Thus I decays at a constant rate.

Duration of effect, for an intravenous dose, is time t when the effect wears off, occurring when the concentration drops below the threshold for effect (Cp). It can be shown that

$$t = \frac{2.303}{k_{el}} \log Cp_0 - \frac{2.303}{k_{el}} \log Cp$$

From this, if Cp_0 is proportional to Qd, a plot of t against the logarithm of the intravenous dose is a straight line with slope $2.303/k_{el}$. From this, doubling the dose increases the duration of action by one half-life.

PART I:
Problems Involving
Drawing a Graph

PROBLEM 1

Statement

The following plasma metoclopramide concentrations were found in a single female patient given a 5-mg intravenous bolus dose:

Time after dose (h)	Concentration (ng/ml)
0 (before dose)	0
0.5	50.0
1	47.0
2	40.0
3	33.0
4	28.0
5	23.0
6	20.0
8	14.5
10	10.0
12	7.2
14	5.3

Draw a graph of the data. Use rectilinear or semilogarithmic coordinates, or both, choosing the coordinates which best display a straight line.

PROBLEM 1

Illustration

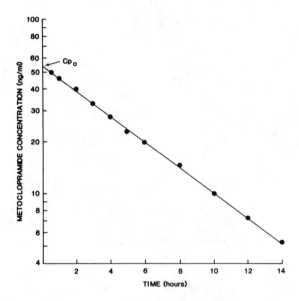

Fig. 1. Graph of metoclopramide concentration against time.

PROBLEM 1

Questions

1.1 What was the order of decay?

    a. Zero   d. Second
    b. 0.5   e. None of the above
    c. First

1.2. What was the rate constant of decay?

    a. $0.22\,h^{-1}$ d. $0.11\,h^{-1}$
    b. $0.17\,h^{-1}$ e. $0.09\,h^{-1}$
    c. $0.13\,h^{-1}$

1.3. Assuming the decay to follow first-order kinetics and assuming answer (b) to be correct in the previous question, what was the half-life of metoclopramide in this patient?

    a. 3.1 h   d. 6.4 h
    b. 4.2 h   e. 7.5 h
    c. 5.3 h

1.4. What was the apparent volume of distribution of metoclopramide in this patient?

    a. 33.0 l   d. 87.6 l
    b. 45.7 l   e. 92.5 l
    c. 65.1 l

1.5. What was the whole body clearance (clearance calculated from plasma level decay) in a patient in whom the first-order half-life was 3.1 h and the apparent volume of distribution was 87.6 l?

    a. 10.3 l/h   d. 27.2 l/h
    b. 15.5 l/h   e. 35.6 l/h
    c. 19.6 l/h

PROBLEM 1

Answers

This group of problems provides an initial exercise concerned with first-order (exponential decay with a constant half-life) kinetics in a one-compartment system.

1.1. . . . .$\boxed{c}$

The graph is a straight line on semilogarithmic coordinates (see Fig. 2 for alternative possibilities).

1.2. . . . .$\boxed{b}$

The rate constant of decay (k_{el}) is obtained from the equation

$$\ln Cp_t = \ln Cp_0 - k_{el}t$$

using a linear regression program or by measuring the half-life from the graph and substituting in

$$k_{el} = \frac{0.693}{T_{1/2}}$$

1.3. . . . .$\boxed{b}$

The half-life from the graph is approximately 4 h. The exact result will vary as a function of artistic skill, but no answer should be less than 3.8 h or greater than 4.6 h.

1.4. . . . .$\boxed{e}$

The apparent volume of distribution (Vd) is obtained from

$$Vd = \frac{Dose}{Cp_0} = \frac{5\,mg}{54\,ng/ml} = 92.5\,l$$

1.5. . . . .$\boxed{c}$

The whole body clearance is given by

$$Cl = Vd\,k_{el}$$

In the case described (not the one in the graph),

$$Cl = 87.6 \times \frac{0.693}{3.1} = 19.6\,l/h$$

PROBLEM 1

Illustration

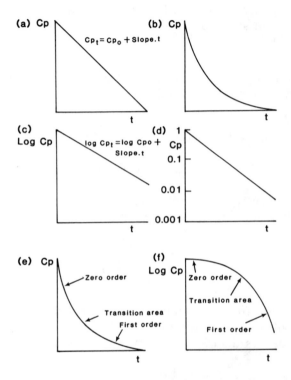

Fig. 2. Model representations of: (a) zero-order decay on rectilinear graph paper; (b) first-order decay on rectilinear graph paper; (c) the graph of (b) plotted as the logarithm of concentration against time on rectilinear graph paper; (d) the graph of (b) plotted as concentrations on semilogarithmic graph paper; (e) the Michaelis–Menten case plotted on rectilinear graph paper; and (f) the Michaelis–Menten case plotted as logarithms of concentration on rectilinear graph paper.

PROBLEM 2

Statement

The following blood ethanol data were obtained from a comatose man on admission (time 0) and at various times after admission.

Time (h)	Concentration (mg / 100 ml)
0	430
1	410
2.5	380
3	370
4	350
6	310
8	270
11	210
14	150

Draw a graph of the data. Use rectilinear or semilogarithmic coordinates, or both, choosing the coordinates which best display a straight line.

PROBLEM 2

Illustration

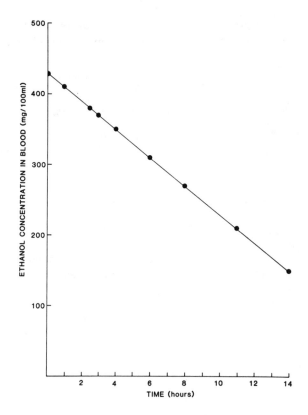

Fig. 3. Graph of ethanol concentration against time.

PROBLEM 2

Questions

2.1. What was the order of decay?

    a. Zero
    b. 0.5
    c. First
    d. Second
    e. None of the above

2.2. Assuming that the body of the patient was a 50-l homogeneous pool, what was the average rate of disappearance of the drug from the whole body during time 1–6 h?

    a. $20 \, \text{mg.h}^{-1}$
    b. $5 \, \text{g.h}^{-1}$
    c. $20 \, \text{mg.100 ml}^{-1}.\text{h}^{-1}$
    d. $0.015\%.\text{h}^{-1}$
    e. $15 \, \text{g.h}^{-1}$

2.3. What was the rate constant of decay in blood?

    a. $20 \, \text{mg.h}^{-1}$
    b. $5 \, \text{g.h}^{-1}$
    c. $20 \, \text{mg.100 ml}^{-1}.\text{h}^{-1}$
    d. $0.015\%.\text{h}^{-1}$
    e. $15 \, \text{g.h}^{-1}$

PROBLEM 2

Answers

2.1. . . . .$\boxed{\text{a}}$

This is an initial exercise in zero-order decay. Zero-order decay is the usual case for ethanol; it also occurs with various drugs at the levels achieved following overdoses. Thus, decay is at a constant rate, shown as a straight line on rectilinear coordinates. This indicates zero-order decay.

2.2. . . . .$\boxed{\text{c}}$

The slope of the graph of the data, drawn on rectilinear coordinates, is given by

$$\frac{410 - 310}{1 - 6} = -\frac{10}{5} = -20\,\text{mg}.100\,\text{ml}^{-1}.\text{h}^{-1}$$

Since the body was equivalent to 50 l of fluid, this could be expressed as:

$$20 \times \frac{50{,}000}{100} = 10{,}000\,\text{mg}.\text{h}^{-1} = 10\,\text{g}.\text{h}^{-1}$$

2.3. . . . .$\boxed{\text{c}}$

In the zero-order case, the rate is equal to the rate constant.

PROBLEM 3

Statement

The following average serum concentrations of tetracycline were obtained following administration of 250 mg capsules of a new generic product and of the recognized standard.

Time	Average serum concentration (μg/ml)	
	Generic	Standard
0.0	0.00	0.00
1.0	0.96	0.99
2.0	1.67	1.69
3.0	1.91	1.96
4.0	1.73	1.92
6.0	1.45	1.80
8.0	1.30	1.55
12.0	1.02	1.15
16.0	0.70	0.83
20.0	0.51	0.61
28.0	0.27	0.32

Graph the data in various ways and select the most suitable coordinates for display of *a straight line in the post-absorptive phase.*

PROBLEM 3

Illustration

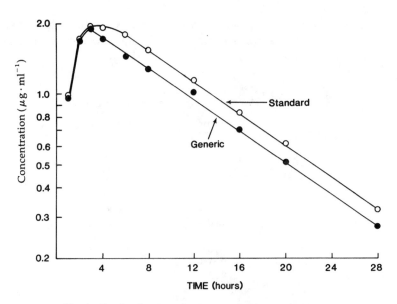

Fig. 4. Graph of tetracycline concentration against time.

PROBLEM 3

Questions

3.1. What is the order of decay in the post-absorptive phase?

 a. Zero   c. First   e. None of the above
 b. 0.5   d. Second

3.2. Calculate the half-life of plasma level decay in the post-absorptive phase for the standard preparation.

 a. 7.0 h   c. 8.0 h   e. 9.0 h
 b. 7.5 h   d. 8.5 h

3.3. Calculate the rate constant of plasma level decay in the post-absorptive phase.

 a. $8.5\,h^{-1}$ c. $0.074\,h^{-1}$ e. $0.082\,h^{-1}$
 b. 8.5 h   d. $0.078\,h^{-1}$

3.4. Calculate the area under the curve from time 0 to infinity for both products and then determine the relative bioavailability (F) of the new generic product. What is the value of F?

 a. 0.76   c. 1.00   e. 1.32
 b. 0.91   d. 1.11

3.5. Calculate t_{max} for the standard preparation.

 a. 3.00 h   c. 4.00 h   e. 6.00 h
 b. 3.72 h   d. 5.10 h

3.6. Calculate C_{max} for the standard preparation.

 a. $2.02\ \mu g.ml^{-1}$ c. $1.97\ \mu g.ml^{-1}$ e. $1.92\ \mu g.ml^{-1}$
 b. $1.82\ \mu g.ml^{-1}$ d. $1.87\ \mu g.ml^{-1}$

PROBLEM 3

Answers

3.1. . . . . $\boxed{c}$

This is an example of a straightforward bioavailability comparison, with requests for some additional information. The graph is a straight line in the post-absorptive (decay) phase when graphed on semilogarithmic graph paper. This indicates first-order decay.

3.2. . . . . $\boxed{d}$

The half-life is 8.5 h, obtained by direct reading from the graph or by applying a linear regression calculation to the logarithms of the data points from 8 to 24 h. Estimates will vary somewhat depending on the accuracy of data fitting and will also vary if data points earlier than 8 h are included.

3.3. . . . . $\boxed{c}$

$$k_{el} = 0.693/8.5 = 0.082 \text{ h}^{-1}$$

The result of this calculation will obviously be wrong if the half-life is wrong. The rate constant can, of course, be obtained from the linear regression calculation and can then be used to calculate the half-life.

3.4. . . . . $\boxed{a}$

The area under the curve for the standard is 30.05 μg·h/ml and that for the new product is 23.20 μg·h/ml. Thus F is 23.20/30.05 = 0.76. Slight variation is seen in these figures as the result of "rounding off" and depending on the value for k_{el}.

3.5. . . . . $\boxed{b}$

Calculation of t_{max} requires prior estimation of k_a. There are several methods for doing this. In this problem there are four data points before the decay phase is established, making use of a method of residuals (feathering) possible. Feathering applied to the "standard" data gives a k_a of 0.63 h^{-1}, so that t_{max} is 3.72 h.

3.6. . . . . $\boxed{e}$

$$Cp = Cp_0[e^{-k_{el}t} - e^{-k_a t}] = 3.0[0.737 - 0.096] = 1.92 \ \mu g/ml$$

where t is 3.72 h, obtained from the previous question.

PROBLEM 4

Statement

Procaine amide was infused into a certain 60-kg patient for 25 hours at a rate of 2 mg/min. The following concentration data were obtained.

A. During infusion	Time (h) from start of infusion	Concentration (μg/ml)
	0	0
	2.5	2.7
	5	3.5
	10	5.1
	15	6.2
	20	6.8
	25	7.0
B. After infusion	Time (h) from end of infusion	Concentration (μg/ml)
	0	7.0
	2	5.1
	4	4.0
	6	3.2
	8	2.3
	10	1.8

Graph the data using either rectilinear or semilogarithmic coordinates. Note that 25 h in A and 0 h in B are the same data point.

PROBLEM 4

Illustration

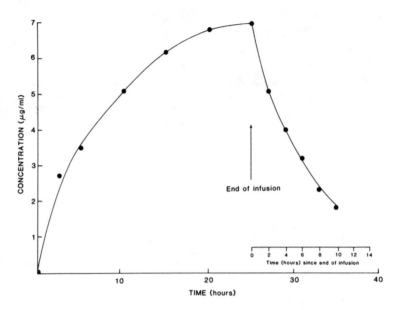

Fig. 5. Graph of procaine amide concentration against time.

PROBLEM 4

Questions

4.1. Calculate the half-life of decay of the drug concentration in plasma once the infusion stopped.

    a. 3.0 h
    b. 4.0 h
    c. 5.0 h
    d. 6.0 h
    e. 7.0 h

4.2. What was the apparent volume of distribution of procaine amide in this patient?

    a. 2.06 l/kg
    b. 1.05 l/kg
    c. 3.07 l/kg
    d. 0.94 l/kg
    e. 4.08 l/kg

4.3. Calculate the concentration of procaine amide at 7.5 h into the infusion

    a. 4.26 μg/ml
    b. 4.51 μg/ml
    c. 4.76 μg/ml
    d. 4.99 μg/ml
    e. 5.24 μg/ml

PROBLEM 4

Answers

4.1. . . . .$\boxed{c}$

This is an example of a standard intravenous infusion. A semilogarithmic graph of the data following the end of the infusion, or application of linear regression to the logarithms of the data, shows the half-life of procaine amide to be 5.0 h.

4.2. . . . .$\boxed{a}$

With a half-life of 5.0 h, 95% of the steady-state concentration is reached in approximately 22 h, so steady state is assumed to be effectively in force during the last 5 hours of the infusion. Accordingly, 7.0 μg/ml can be taken as Cp_{ss} in

$$Cp_{ss} = k_0/Vd \cdot k_{el}$$

where k_0 is the infusion rate, Vd is the apparent volume of distribution, and $k_{el} = 0.693/T_{1/2}$. Thus

$$Vd = 2 \times 60/(7.0 \times 0.693/5.0) = 123.7 \, l$$

or 2.06 l/kg.

4.3. . . . .$\boxed{b}$

This is given by

$$Cp_t = k_0/Vd \cdot k_{el}[1 - e^{-k_{el}t}]$$

where t is 7.5 h. $Cp_t = 4.51$ μg/ml, using $k_{el} = 0.1386 \, h^{-1}$ ($= 0.693/5.0$), agreeing with the conclusion likely from visual inspection of the graph. There is an equation which treats both sections of the data at the same time:

$$Cp_t = \frac{k_0}{Vd \cdot k_{el}} [(1 - e^{-k_{el}t_l})(e^{-k_{el}(t - t_l)})]$$

where t_l is infusion time and t is time since the start of the infusion. This is useful for simulation, but it does not obviate the need for evaluation of k_{el}.

PROBLEM 5

Statement

The following concentrations (in ng/ml) of clonidine were recorded in a 65-kg patient given single i.v. (0.1 mg) and oral (0.2 mg) doses of the drug one month apart:

Time after dose (h)	1	2	4	8	12
I.V. dose	0.69	0.61	0.52	0.34	0.22
Oral dose	0.50	0.78	0.78	0.49	0.33

At a later date, the patient was treated with a transdermal preparation designed to deliver 0.1 mg/day for one week; the mean steady-state clonidine concentration recorded during transdermal dosing was 0.33 ng/ml. You may assume in answering the following questions that a one-compartment model is applicable, that there were no changes in clonidine pharmacokinetics between the doses, and that none of the processes involved show dose-dependency.

Draw a graph of the oral and i.v. dose data on one sheet of either rectilinear or semilogarithmic graph paper.

PROBLEM 5

Illustration

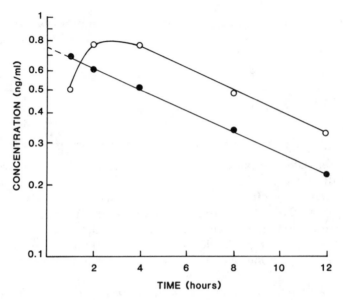

Fig. 6. Graph of clonidine concentration against time.

PROBLEM 5

Questions

5.1. Calculate the half-life of clonidine following the intraveneous dose.

    a. 5.5 h   c. 7.5 h   e. 9.5 h
    b. 6.5 h   d. 8.5 h

5.2. Calculate the apparent volume of distribution of clonidine.

    a. 1.0 l/kg   c. 2.0 l/kg   e. 3.0 l/kg
    b. 1.5 l/kg   d. 2.5 l/kg

5.3. Calculate the total body clearance (calculated from plasma level decay) of clonidine in a patient in whom 8.0 h is the half-life and 2.0 l/kg is the apparent volume of distribution.

    a. 173 ml.min^{-1}.kg^{-1} d. 2.9 ml.min^{-1}.kg^{-1}
    b. 290 ml.min^{-1}.kg^{-1} e. 0.173 ml.min^{-1}.kg^{-1}
    c. 2.9 ml.min^{-1}

5.4. Calculate the bioavailability (F) of oral clonidine.

    a. 0.33   c. 0.61   e. 0.90
    b. 0.19   d. 1.56

5.5. Calculate the bioavailability of transdermal clonidine in the patient, assuming that answers (b) in question 5.1 and (c) in question 5.2 are correct.

    a. 1.2   c. 0.8   e. 1.1
    b. 1.0   d. 0.9

5.6. Assuming that the correct answer to question 5.3 was 2.9 ml.min^{-1}.kg^{-1} and that the elimination of clonidine consists solely of hepatic metabolism *plus* renal excretion of unmetabolized drug, calculate the hepatic clearance given that the renal clearance is 2.0 ml.min^{-1}.kg^{-1}.

    a. 0.65 ml.min^{-1}.kg^{-1} d. 5.10 ml.min^{-1}.kg^{-1}
    b. −1.10 ml.min^{-1}.kg^{-1} e. 1.55 ml.min^{-1}.kg^{-1}
    c. 0.90 ml.min^{-1}.kg^{-1}

PROBLEM 5

Answers

5.1. . . . .$\boxed{b}$

The half-life is obtained by direct reading from the semilogarithmic graph or by means of linear regression; it is approximately 6.5 h, but definitely not 5.5 or 7.5 h.

5.2. . . . .$\boxed{c}$

The volume of distribution (Vd) is given by

$$Vd = Dose/Cp_0$$

where Cp_0 is the intercept of the intravenous dose graph on the y-axis. In this case $Vd = 0.1 \times 1000 \times 1000/0.76$ ml $= 132{,}000$ ml or 2.0 l/kg.

5.3. . . . .$\boxed{d}$

Total body clearance (Cl_{TOT}) is defined by

$$Cl_{TOT} = Vd \cdot k_{el} = 2.0 \times \frac{0.693}{8.0}\ l.kg^{-1}.h^{-1} = 0.173\ l.kg^{-1}.h^{-1}$$

This is not one of the possible answers, but it is the same as 2.9 ml/kg/min.

5.4. . . . .$\boxed{c}$

This requires calculation of the area under the curves (AUC) of the two doses and correction for the dose differences. Thus,

$$\text{I.V. dose: AUC} = Cp_0 \Big/ \frac{0.693}{T_{1/2}} = \frac{0.76 \times 6.5}{0.693} = 7.13\ ng \cdot h/ml$$

Oral dose: AUC computed by means of
the trapezoidal rule $= 8.69$

$$F = \frac{8.69/0.2}{7.13/0.1} = 0.61$$

This calculation is heavily dependent on estimates of Cp_0 and

$T_{1/2}$, but no calculation should result in an F beyond the limits of 0.5 and 0.7.

5.5. . . . .$\boxed{e}$

This requires the realization that transdermal treatment for a week can be treated as an application of steady state, so that

$$Cp_{ss} = k_0/Vd \cdot k_{el}$$

as in other questions. In this case

$$Cp_{ss} = \frac{0.1}{24} \times 1000 \left/ 65 \times 2.0 \times \frac{0.693}{0.5} \right.$$

in which Cp_{ss} is the expected steady-state concentration with a volume of distribution of 2.0 l/kg and a half-life of 6.5 h. From this, $Cp_{ss} = 0.30$ ng/ml, so the recorded Cp_{ss} was 10% higher than expected, giving $F = 1.1$. At first this seems nonsensical, but it may have resulted from the presence of a small loading dose of clonidine in the adhesive of the transdermal preparation.

5.6. . . . .$\boxed{c}$

Clearances are additive, so that

$$Cl_{TOT} = \text{Renal clearance} + \text{Hepatic clearance}$$

Hence

$$2.9 = 2.0 + \text{Hepatic clearance}$$

$$\text{Hepatic clearance} = 2.9 - 2.0 \ \text{ml.min}^{-1}.\text{kg}^{-1} = 0.9 \ \text{ml.min}^{-1}.\text{kg}^{-1}$$

PROBLEM 6

Statement

The following data were recorded for the decline in concentration of phenobarbital in the plasma of a 92-kg patient who had taken an overdose of the drug:

Time since dose (days)	Concentration ($\mu g \cdot ml^{-1}$)
0.5	86.5
1.0	83.0
2.0	76.0
3.0	70.5
4.0	66.0
6.0	53.6
8.0	43.4
12.0	24.5
18.0	7.5
20.0	5.0
24.0	2.2
28.0	1.0

Graph the data using both semilogarithmic and rectilinear coordinates. Note that the data accords with Michaelis–Menten decay.

PROBLEM 6

Illustration

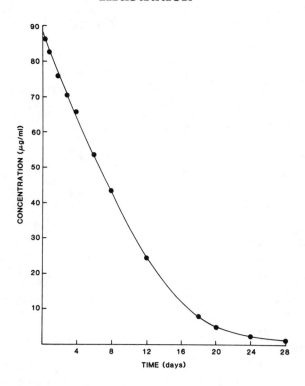

Fig. 7. Graph of phenobarbital concentration against time (rectilinear coordinates).

PROBLEM 6

Illustration

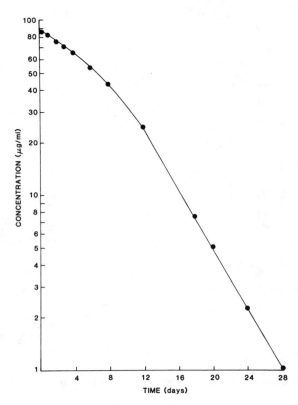

Fig. 8. Graph of phenobarbital concentration against time (semilogarithmic coordinates).

PROBLEM 6

Questions

6.1. What was the recorded V_{max} in units of rate of change of concentration in plasma?

    a. $5.0 \ \mu g.ml^{-1}.day^{-1}$ d. $9.0 \ \mu g.ml^{-1}.day^{-1}$
    b. $8.0 \ \mu g.ml^{-1}.day^{-1}$ e. $7.0 \ \mu g.ml^{-1}.day^{-1}$
    c. $6.0 \ \mu g.ml^{-1}.day^{-1}$

6.2. What was the first-order rate constant for plasma level decay in later stages of the investigation?

    a. $0.075 \ days^{-1}$ c. $0.15 \ days^{-1}$ e. $0.10 \ days^{-1}$
    b. $0.05 \ days^{-1}$ d. $0.20 \ days^{-1}$

6.3. What was the K_m for phenobarbital elimination in the patient for whom $6.0 \ \mu g.ml^{-1}.day^{-1}$ was the correct answer in question 6.1 and for whom $0.2 \ days^{-1}$ was the correct answer in question 6.2?

    a. $30.0 \ \mu g/ml$ c. $35.0 \ \mu g/ml$ e. $40.0 \ \mu g/ml$
    b. $32.5 \ \mu g/ml$ d. $37.5 \ \mu g/ml$

6.4. The apparent volume of distribution (Vd) of phenobarbital is $0.88 \ 1/kg$. What was the approximate dose in the patient from whom the data in the table was collected?

    a. $13.0 \ g$ c. $8.5 \ g$ e. $6.5 \ g$
    b. $10.1 \ g$ d. $7.3 \ g$

6.5. The same patient as in questions 6.1, 6.2, and 6.4 was later found to have a k_{el} for phenobarbital of $0.2 \ days^{-1}$. He was then prescribed 300 mg/day of phenobarbital. His steady-state concentration after three weeks of treatment was $14.8 \ \mu g/ml$. By how much was this less than would have been predicted on the basis of first-order kinetics alone?

    a. $3.7 \ \mu g/ml$ c. $12.0 \ \mu g/ml$ e. $18.5 \ \mu g/ml$
    b. $9.9 \ \mu g/ml$ d. $14.8 \ \mu g/ml$

PROBLEM 6

Answers

6.1. . . . . $\boxed{c}$

This example illustrates the various features of a Michaelis–Menten decay. V_{max} is obtained from the top left, straight part of the graph on rectilinear coordinates; it is the slope from time 0.5 to no greater than 4 days.

$$\text{Slope} = \frac{86.5 - 66}{0.5 - 4} = -5.85 \ \mu\text{g.ml}^{-1}.\text{day}^{-1}$$

Linear regression of all data from 0.5–4 days gives 5.91 μg.ml^{-1}.day^{-1}. Use of less data gives slope values ranging up to 7.0 μg.ml^{-1}.day^{-1}. The negative sign is redundant in expressing a rate of change.

6.2. . . . . $\boxed{d}$

The half-life in the later stages (12–28 days) was 3.5 days, obtained from visual inspection of the semilogarithmic graph or from linear regression. Thus $k_{el} = 0.693/3.5 = 0.2$ days^{-1}.

6.3. . . . . $\boxed{a}$

$k_{el} = V_{max}/K_m$

So: $K_m = V_{max}/k_{el} = \dfrac{6.0}{0.2} = 30.0 \ \mu\text{g/ml}$

6.4. . . . . $\boxed{d}$

$\text{Vd} = \text{Dose}/\text{Cp}_0$

$\text{Dose} = \text{Vd} \times \text{Cp}_0 = 0.88 \times 92 \times 90 \times \dfrac{1}{1000} = 7.3 \ \text{g}$

6.5. . . . . $\boxed{a}$

$\text{Cp}_{ss} = k_0/\text{Vd} \cdot k_{el} = \dfrac{300}{0.88 \times 92 \times 0.2} = 18.53 \ \mu\text{g/ml}$

$18.53 - 14.8 = 3.7 \ \mu\text{g/ml}$

PROBLEM 7

Statement

The following plasma concentration data were collected in a single 66.7 kg male subject given a 30 mg/kg dose of sulfamethazine.

Time since dose (h)	Concentration (μg/ml)	
	Sulfamethazine	Acetylsulfamethazine
0	0	0
0.25	14	2
0.5	22	5
1	33	14
1.5	44	25
2	43	33
3	40	42
4	30	47
5	23	48
6	18	45
8	11	41
12	4	35
21	—	24
26	—	19

Draw a graph of concentration vs. time on either linear or semilogarithmic coordinates.

PROBLEM 7

Illustration

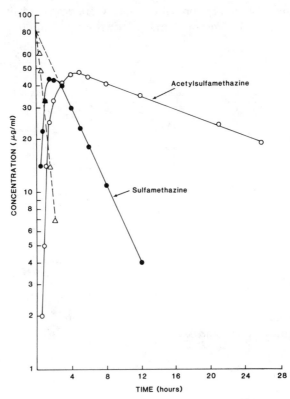

Fig. 9. Graph of sulfamethazine and acetylsulfamethazine concentration against time.

PROBLEM 7

Questions

7.1. Calculate the half-life of sulfamethazine once the maximum was passed.

    a. 2.0 h   c. 3.5 h   e. 4.5 h
    b. 2.8 h   d. 4.0 h

7.2. Calculate the rate constant of absorption for sulfamethazine.

    a. $0.6\,h^{-1}$ c. $1.4\,h^{-1}$ e. $2.8\,h^{-1}$
    b. $0.9\,h^{-1}$ d. $2.0\,h^{-1}$

7.3. Calculate the renal clearance of sulfamethazine given the following additional information; the volume of urine from 6–8 h post-dosage was 132 ml and the concentration of sulfamethazine in this urine sample was 70 $\mu g/ml$.

    a. 646.1 ml/min   c. 5.4 ml/h   e. $0.9\,h^{-1}$
    b. 120.0 ml/min   d. 5.4 ml/min

7.4. Calculate the renal clearance of acetylsulfamethazine given that the acetylsulfamethazine concentration in the same sample as in the previous question was 2495 $\mu g/ml$.

    a. 63.8 ml/min   c. 63.8 ml/h   e. 191.9 ml/min
    b. 7659.1 ml/min   d. 5.4 ml/min

7.5. Assuming that the following model accounts for *all* sulfamethazine elimination,

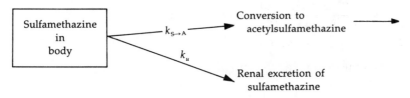

estimate $k_{S \to A}$ given that the bioavailability (F) of sulfamethazine is unity and that the apparent volume of distribution is 0.15 l/kg.

    a. $0.032\,h^{-1}$ c. $0.280\,h^{-1}$ e. $0.216\,h^{-1}$
    b. $0.248\,h^{-1}$ d. $0.496\,h^{-1}$

PROBLEM 7

Answers

7.1. . . . .$\boxed{\text{b}}$

Reading from the graph, or by linear regression of log Cp_t vs. t, the half-life is 2.8 h. The estimate depends on whether relatively early points such as that at 3 h are used, but no estimate should be less than 2.5 h or greater than 3.1 h.

7.2. . . . .$\boxed{\text{c}}$

From the method of residuals line (open triangles), the half-life of absorption is 0.5 h, so that

$$k_a = 0.693 / 0.5 = 1.136 \, \text{h}^{-1}$$

7.3. . . . .$\boxed{\text{d}}$

Clearance (Cl) = UV/P

where U is urinary concentration, V is urinary flow rate, and P is midpoint plasma concentration during the urine collection period.

$$Cl = \frac{70 \times 132 / 120}{14.3} = 5.4 \, \text{ml/min}$$

(Note that 14.3 is the concentration halfway between 6 and 8 hours.)

7.4. . . . .$\boxed{\text{a}}$

$$Cl = \frac{2495 \times 132 / 120}{43} = 63.8 \, \text{ml/min}$$

7.5. . . . .$\boxed{\text{e}}$

Renal clearance = 5.4 ml/min

$$Cl = Vd \cdot k_u$$

$$k_u = Cl/Vd = 5.4 \times 60 / 0.15 \times 66.7 \times 1000 = 0.032 \, \text{h}^{-1}$$

$$k_{el} = k_u + k_{S \to A}$$

$$\frac{0.693}{2.8} = 0.032 + k_{S \to A}$$

$$k_{S \to A} = 0.216 \, \text{h}^{-1}$$

PROBLEM 8

Statement

Scopolamine can be administered intravenously or by means of transdermal "skin patches" (as well as by means of tablets or i.m.). The following urine scopolamine concentration/volume data were obtained in a single subject treated with a continuous i.v. infusion (I) and with a skin patch (II) on separate occasions (administration was for 3 days in each case):

Dose/measure	Time after initiation of dose (h)							
	0–12	12–24	24–48	48–72	72–75	75–78	78–81	81–84
I/urine volume (ml)	720	616	1200	953	221	150	180	200
I/drug concentration in urine (ng/ml)	6.7	8.4	8.4	10.8	3.1	0.38	0.047	0.0056
II/urine volume (ml)	655	1900	1900	1000	231	200	190	201
II/drug concentration in urine (ng/ml)	6.6	6.3	6.6	12.7	6.0	3.6	2.5	0.90

Draw a graph of renal excretion rate vs. time for both doses using either semilogarithmic or rectilinear coordinates.

PROBLEM 8

Illustration

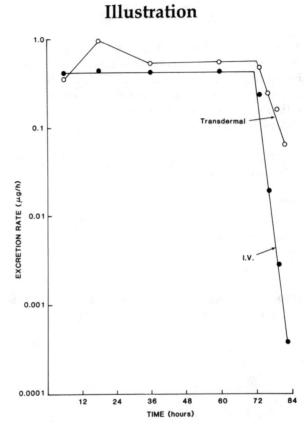

Fig. 10. Graph of scopolamine excretion rate against time.

PROBLEM 8

Questions

8.1. Calculate the half-life of decay of the rate of urinary drug excretion rate with time once the i.v. infusion was stopped.

   a. 0.5 h
   b. 1.0 h
   c. 1.5 h
   d. 2.0 h
   e. 2.5 h

8.2. Assuming constant renal clearance, what was the half-life in plasma once the i.v. infusion was stopped?

   a. 0.5 h
   b. 1.0 h
   c. 1.5 h
   d. 2.0 h
   e. 2.5 h

8.3. Given that the i.v. infusion was at a rate of 0.8 mg/day, use the urinary excretion data to estimate the rate of delivery from the skin patch.

   a. 0.6 mg/day
   b. 0.8 mg/day
   c. 1.0 mg/day
   d. 1.2 mg/day
   e. 1.4 mg/day

8.4. Given that the plasma level was 0.1 ng/ml at the midpoint of the 24–48 h collection period during the i.v. infusion, calculate the renal clearance of scopolamine.

   a. 70 ml/min
   b. 120 ml/min
   c. 240 ml/min
   d. 510 ml/min
   e. 700 ml/min

PROBLEM 8

Answers

8.1. . . . .$\boxed{\text{b}}$

It is not always appreciated that a rate of change can itself change with time. When the renal clearance is constant, the rate of change of excretion rate reflects changes in the concentration in plasma. The validity of the 1.0-h half-life determination is self-explanatory.

8.2. . . . .$\boxed{\text{b}}$

If renal clearance is constant, the renal excretion rate is proportional to concentration in plasma, so that the half-life of decay of the renal excretion rate is equal to the half-life of decay of the concentrations in plasma.

8.3. . . . .$\boxed{\text{c}}$

Steady-state conditions apply with the plasma concentration so the renal excretion rate is proportional to the input rate. For the patch dose, the mean excretion rate equals 0.525 μg/h, while the mean excretion rate following the i.v. dose is 0.425 μg/h. Hence the input for the patch dose is given by

$$\text{Input rate} = \frac{0.8 \times 0.525}{0.425} = 1\,\text{mg/day}$$

8.4. . . . .$\boxed{\text{a}}$

$$Cl_R = UV/P$$

$$= \frac{8.4 \times \dfrac{1200}{12}}{0.1}$$

$$= 8400\,\text{ml/h}$$

$$= 700\,\text{ml/min}$$

PROBLEM 9

Statement

A patient on phenytoin was dosed on four different occasions, with different phenytoin doses, to steady state. His doses and plasma concentrations were:

Daily dose (mg)	Concentration in plasma (Cp_{ss}) ($\mu g/ml$)
300	5.3
400	9.2
500	16.3
600	35.0

Draw a straight-line graph relating this data.

PROBLEM 9

Illustration

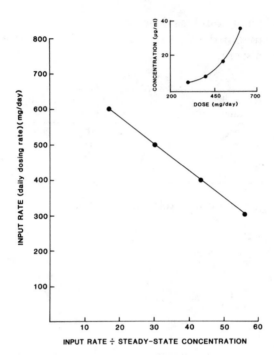

Fig. 11. Graph of phenytoin dosing rate against dosing rate divided by steady-state concentration (inset: concentration against dose for the same data).

PROBLEM 9

Questions

9.1. Calculate the apparent K_m for this patient.

    a. 5.3 μg/ml
    b. 7.7 μg/ml
    c. 9.2 μg/ml
    d. 16.3 μg/ml
    e. 35.0 μg/ml

9.2. Calculate the V_{max} for this patient.

    a. 450 μg/ml
    b. 35.0 μg/ml
    c. 600 mg/day
    d. 731 mg/day
    e. 900 ng/day

9.3. Consider a hypothetical situation in which only the 300- and 400-mg doses had been studied and a linear extrapolation assuming Cp_{ss} to be directly proportional to daily dose had been used to predict the dose required to induce a concentration in plasma of 15 μg/ml. By how much would the prediction have been wrong?

    a. 21.77 μg/ml too high
    b. 15.00 μg/ml too low
    c. 57 mg/day too high
    d. 57 mg/day too low
    e. No error

PROBLEM 9

Answers

9.1. . . . .$\boxed{b}$

The straight-line relationship is

$$\text{Dosing rate } (k_0) = V_{\max} - K_m \frac{\text{Dosing rate } (k_0)}{\text{Steady-state conc. } (Cp_{ss})}$$

The slope is negative, so that K_m is positive (7.7 μg/ml).

9.2. . . . .$\boxed{c}$

$V_{\max}$ is equal to the intercept on the y-axis (731 mg/day).

9.3. . . . .$\boxed{c}$

Linear extrapolation of the two lower data points would have predicted a dose of 540 mg/day to give 15 μg/ml. In fact, this would have given 21.77 μg/ml, from

$$Cp_{ss} = \frac{K_m \times k_0}{V_{\max} - k_0}$$

The prediction would have been wrong in overestimating the dose such that Cp_{ss} would have been 6.77 μg/ml too high. The dose which would result in a plasma concentration of 15 μg/ml is given by

$$k_0 = \frac{V_{\max} \times Cp_{ss}}{K_m + Cp_{ss}}$$

which equals 483 mg in this case, so the prediction of 540 mg/day would have been 57 mg/day too high.

PROBLEM 10

Statement

A 45-kg patient dosed with gentamicin had the following plasma levels recorded after receiving his initial dose of 60 mg over 30 minutes.

Time since end of infusion (min)	Concentration (μg/ml)
0	12.0
0.25	8.0
0.50	5.8
0.75	5.2
1.0	5.0
3.0	4.3
7.0	2.2
9.0	1.8

Draw a graph of the data using semilogarithmic coordinates.

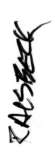

PROBLEM 10

Illustration

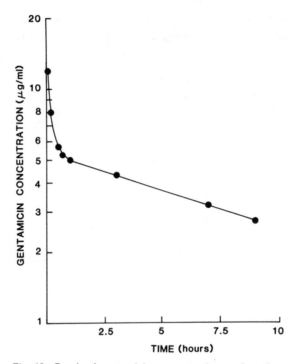

Fig. 12. Graph of gentamicin concentration against time.

PROBLEM 10

Questions

10.1. Calculate the rate constant of decline of plasma concentration in the β-phase of plasma level decay.

    a. $0.032\,h^{-1}$
    b. $0.043\,h^{-1}$
    c. $0.054\,h^{-1}$
    d. $0.065\,h^{-1}$
    e. $0.076\,h^{-1}$

10.2. Calculate α in the equation: $Cp_t = Ae^{-\alpha t} + Be^{-\beta t}$

    a. $0.50\,h^{-1}$
    b. $1.75\,h^{-1}$
    c. $1.00\,h^{-1}$
    d. $1.50\,h^{-1}$
    e. $1.25\,h^{-1}$

10.3. Calculate the apparent volume of distribution (Vd) of gentamicin from the equation:

$$Vd = Vd(\text{extrapol.}) = Dose/B$$

    a. $0.15\,l/kg$
    b. $0.20\,l/kg$
    c. $0.25\,l/kg$
    d. $0.30\,l/kg$
    e. $0.35\,l/kg$

10.4. Assuming that (i) the β-phase extends with the same kinetics until at least the 24-h point; (ii) concentrations 1-h post infusion are desirably 7.5 $\mu g/ml$ or above; and (iii) troughs (concentrations just before subsequent doses) should be below 20 $\mu g/ml$, calculate a convenient dosage regimen.

    a. 100 mg every 24 h
    b. 60 mg every 8 h
    c. 90 mg every 8 h
    d. 60 mg every 24 h
    e. 90 mg every 20 h

PROBLEM 10

Answers

10.1. . . . .$\boxed{e}$

Gentamicin is a multi-compartment drug which is often treated as a single-compartment example. The plasma levels decay rapidly at first (α-phase) and then more slowly (β-phase). Standard techniques lead to the conclusion that the rate constant of decay in the β-phase is $0.076\,h^{-1}$.

10.2. . . . .$\boxed{b}$

This requires a "feathering" or method of residuals analysis. However, there is such a sharp demarcation between the two phases (fast and slow) that the data from 0 to 0.5 h is almost coincident with the α-phase construction line. It is self-evident that the concentration in the first 30 minutes falls with a half-life of less than 0.5 h and so with a rate constant of more than $1.5\,h^{-1}$.

10.3. . . . .$\boxed{c}$

$$Vd(\text{extrapol.}) = \frac{60}{45} \times \frac{1}{5.3} = 0.25\,l/kg$$

10.4. . . . .$\boxed{a}$

The dose must be raised by at least 50% to cause peaks of at least 7.5 μg/ml. If the dose is increased to 90 mg, then the concentration at 8 h becomes approximately 45 μg/ml. It is thus necessary to extend the dosing interval. It can be calculated that a 90-mg dose will give 2 μg/ml or less at 20 h, but this is an inconvenient dosing interval; 100 mg every 24 h ensures peaks above 7.5 μg/ml, troughs 2 μg/ml or below, and a convenient dosing interval of 24 h.

PROBLEM 11

Statement

The following concentrations of lithium were obtained following a single test dose of lithium carbonate in a single individual:

Time after dose (h)	Concentration (mEq/l)
0	0
0.5	0.26
1.0	0.65
1.5	0.67
2.0	0.65
3.0	0.61
4.0	0.57
5.0	0.53
6.0	0.49
8.0	0.43

Graph the data on semilogarithmic or rectilinear coordinates.

PROBLEM 11

Illustration

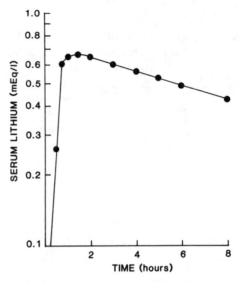

Fig. 13. Graph of lithium concentration against time.

PROBLEM 11

Questions

11.1. Calculate the half-life of lithium in the post-absorptive phase of the investigation.

    a. 6 h
    b. 7 h
    c. 8 h
    d. 9 h
    e. 10 h

11.2. If the same dose was given every eight hours for 2–3 weeks, such that a pseudo-steady state comprising a repeating pattern of peaks and troughs was reached, what would be the trough level?

    a. 0.91 mEq/l
    b. 1.01 mEq/l
    c. 1.13 mEq/l
    d. 1.24 mEq/l
    e. 1.35 mEq/l

11.3. How would you describe the fluctuation between peaks and troughs in the pseudo-steady state?

    a. 100% increases followed by 100% falls
    b. 100% increases followed by 63.5% falls
    c. 57.4% fluctuation
    d. 36.5% fluctuation
    e. 57.4% increases followed by 36.5% falls

PROBLEM 11

Answers

11.1. . . . . $\boxed{e}$

Lithium has no metabolites, so the serum concentration decay is caused by renal excretion. The calculation of a 10-h half-life follows from standard approaches.

11.2. . . . . $\boxed{b}$

This is obtained from

$$Cp_{ss}^{min} = \frac{Cp_{first\ dose}^{min}}{1 - e^{-Kt}} = \frac{0.43}{1 - e^{-(0.693/10)\cdot 8}} = \frac{0.43}{0.4255} = 1.01 \text{ mEq}/l$$

11.3. . . . . $\boxed{e}$

The figure 0.4255 in the previous problem is a proportionality factor representing the proportional fall from C_p (the theoretical, extrapolated concentration at $t = 0$ after the first dose) to the trough. It can be applied to the peak occurring at 1.5 h just as easily as to the trough. Thus

$$Cp_{ss}^{max} = \frac{0.67}{0.4255} = 1.59$$

$\qquad$ = the maximum at 1.5 h after the dose at steady state.

In this situation, the fluctuation between maximum and minimum at steady state will be between 1.59 and 1.01, and will involve 57.4% increases and 36.5% decreases.

PART II:
Single Answer
Calculation
Problems

PROBLEM 12

Log_{10} of 10 is:

    a. 0.693
    b. 2.303
    c. 1.0
    d. 22,026.5
    e. 1×10^{10}

Answer . . . .$\boxed{c}$

PROBLEM 13

The natural logarithm of 10 is:

    a. 0.693
    b. 2.303
    c. 1.0
    d. 22,026.5
    e. 1×10^{10}

Answer . . . .$\boxed{b}$

PROBLEM 14

The natural logarithm of 20 is:

    a. 4.8×10^{8}
    b. 1.3
    c. 10×10^{19}
    d. 400
    e. 3.0

Answer . . . .$\boxed{e}$

PROBLEM 15

The value of exp (-0.4×5) is:

    a. 0.135
    b. 7.4
    c. 0
    d. 1×10^{20}
    e. 400

Answer . . . .$\boxed{a}$

PROBLEM 16

The slope of a two-point graph in which the data points are (1) $y = 10, x = 1$ and (2) $y = 6$, $x = 3$ is:

    a. -1
    b. -2
    c. -3
    d. -4
    e. -5

Answer . . . .$\boxed{b}$

PROBLEM 17

The slope of a line defined by the equation $\ln Cp_t = \ln Cp_0 - 0.1\, t$ is:

    a. 10
    b. $\ln 10$
    c. 0.1
    d. -0.1
    e. $0.1\, t$

Answer . . . .$\boxed{d}$

PROBLEM 18

Calculate the regression coefficient for the following data: $t = 0$, $Cp = 20$; $t = 1.5$, $Cp = 14.3$; $t = 3.5$, $Cp = 6.7$; $t = 3.5$, $Cp = 6.7$; $t = 5$, $Cp = 1$ (Cp in mg/l; t in h).

    a. $6.0 \, mg.l^{-1}.h^{-1}$
    b. $4.9 \, mg.l^{-1}.h^{-1}$
    c. $3.8 \, mg.l^{-1}.h^{-1}$
    d. $2.7 \, ml.l^{-1}.h^{-1}$
    e. $1.6 \, mg.l^{-1}.h^{-1}$

Answer . . . . $\boxed{c}$

PROBLEM 19

Apply the trapezoidal rule to calculate the area under the curve from 1 to 60 min from the following data:

Time (min)	Concentration ($\mu g/ml$)
0	0
10	0.6
20	1.3
30	0.5
40	0.1
60	0.05

    a. $2.6 \, \mu g.min/ml$
    b. $25.25 \, \mu g.min/ml$
    c. $26.0 \, \mu g.min/ml$
    d. $0.26 \, \mu g.h/ml$
    e. $0.52 \, \mu g.h/ml$

Answer . . . . $\boxed{c}$

$$[AUC]_{t_{n-1}}^{t} = \frac{C_{n-1} + C_n}{2} (t_n - t_{n-1})$$

Thus:

$$0\text{--}10: \frac{0 + 0.6}{2}(10 - 0) = 3.0$$

$$10\text{--}20: \frac{0.6 + 1.3}{2}(20 - 10) = 9.5$$

$$20\text{--}30: \frac{1.3 + 0.5}{2}(30 - 20) = 9.0$$

$$30\text{--}40: \frac{0.5 + 0.1}{2}(40 - 30) = 3.0$$

$$40\text{--}60: \frac{0.1 + 0.05}{2}(60 - 40) = 1.5$$

$$3.0 + 9.5 + 9.0 + 3.0 + 1.5 = 26.0 \ \mu g \cdot \min/ml$$

PROBLEM 20

Calculate the rate constant of ethanol elimination in a driver who had the following blood ethanol concentrations measured: on arrest, 160 mg/100 ml; one hour later, 142 mg/100 ml; three hours after arrest, 106 mg/100 ml; six hours after arrest 52 mg/100 ml. Assume an apparent volume of distribution of 50 l.

    a. 18 mg/h
    b. 9 mg.kg^{-1}.h^{-1}
    c. 4.5 g/h
    d. 9 g/h
    e. 36 mg.kg^{-1}.h^{-1}

Answer . . . .$\boxed{d}$

This requires the knowledge that ethanol concentrations in plasma decay at a constant rate (zero-order kinetics); this can be verified by inspection of the concentration data given. In zero-order cases, the rate and the rate constant are identical (contrast first-order cases). In this example, the rate of decline in concentration is $(160 - 142)/1$ or $(160 - 106)/2$ or $(106 - 52)/3$, etc., which is 18 mg.100 ml^{-1}.h^{-1}. Since the volume of distribution is 50 l and 18 mg.100 ml^{-1}.h^{-1} is not given as a possible correct answer, answer (d) is the correct one, from:

$$\text{Rate constant} = 18 \times \frac{50}{100} \times 1000 = 9000 \ mg/h = 9 \ g/h$$

PROBLEM 21

In an overdose patient weighing 70 kg, phenobarbital concentrations were measured on admission and five hours later as 90 μg/ml and 63 μg/ml. The apparent volume of distribution was 1 l/kg. Calculate the zero-order rate of elimination of phenobarbital in this patient.

    a. 70 kg/h
    b. 10 mg.l^{-1}.h^{-1}
    c. 378 mg/h
    d. 378 mg.l^{-1}.h^{-1}
    e. 5.4 mg/h

Answer . . . .$\boxed{c}$

$$\text{Rate} = \frac{90 - 63}{5} \times 70 \times 1$$

$$= 378 \text{ mg/h}$$

PROBLEM 22

A drug was delivered intravenously into a one-compartment system of volume 50 l at a dose of 1 mg. After one hour, ln Cp_t, with Cp_t measured in ng/ml, was 2.7085. What was the half-life of the drug in the system, assuming exponential decay?

    a. 0.2872 h^{-1}
    b. 0.365
    c. 17.2 min
    d. 0.5744 h
    e. 2.4129 h

Answer . . . .$\boxed{e}$

This is a straightforward first-order decay problem, except that the unknown is the half-life, rather than the more usual Cp_t at a given t with Cp_0 and k_{el} (or $T_{1/2}$) given.

$$Cp_0 = 0.02 \text{ mg}/l = 20 \text{ ng}/\text{ml}$$

$$\ln Cp_t = \ln Cp_0 - k_{el}t$$

$$2.7085 = 2.9957 - k_{el}t$$

$$t = 1$$

$$k_{el} = 0.2872$$

$$T_{1/2} = 0.693/0.2872 = 2.4129 \text{ h}$$

PROBLEM 23

What was the systematic clearance (clearance calculated from plasma level decay) in a 52.7 kg patient for whom the correct answer in the previous question was 0.5744 h? Vd = 1 l/kg.

a. $63.6 \text{ l.kg}^{-1}.\text{h}^{-1}$
b. $1.273 \text{ l.kg}^{-1}.\text{h}^{-1}$
c. $0.2872 \text{ l.kg}^{-1}.\text{h}^{-1}$
d. 14.36 l/h
e. $0.0414 \text{ l.kg}^{-1}.\text{min}^{-1}$

Answer . . . . [a]

$$Vd = 1 \text{ l/kg}$$

$$Wt. = 52.7 \text{ kg}$$

$$Cl = Vd \cdot k_{el} = 52.7 \times 1 \times \frac{0.693}{0.5744} = 63.6 \text{ l.kg}^{-1}.\text{h}^{-1}$$

PROBLEM 24

Calculate the half-life of theophylline in a patient from whom the following data were collected: first data point, 22 μg/ml; 0.5 h later, 21.04 μg/ml; 2 h after first data point, 18.4 μg/ml; 4 h after first data point, 15.4 μg/ml.

 a. 5.0 h
 b. 6.9 h
 c. 7.8 h
 d. 8.7 h
 e. 9.6 h

Answer . . . .$\boxed{c}$

Examination of the data, the request for half-life calculation, and knowledge of theophylline tells us that a first-order model is appropriate. Linear regression analysis fitting the data to the model represented by the equation

$$\ln Cp_t = \ln Cp_0 - k_{el}t$$

leads to the conclusion that k_{el} is 0.089 h^{-1}. Since

$$T_{1/2} = 0.693 / k_{el}$$

the half-life is 7.8 h.

PROBLEM 25

Calculate the apparent volume of distribution of theophylline in the patient of the previous question, given the added information that the first data point was one hour after the end of an infusion dose of theophylline and that the correct half-life was 7.8 h. The total body content of theophylline at the end of the infusion was 600 mg.

 a. 23.85 l
 b. 24.96 l
 c. 26.01 l
 d. 27.12 l
 e. 28.23 l

Answer . . . .$\boxed{b}$

The equation which describes the decay of plasma theophylline concentration with time is

$$Cp_t = Cp_0 \exp(-k_{el}t)$$

The question requires calculation of the concentration one hour *before* the first determined concentration (an unusual request), so:

$$x = 22 \exp\left(-\frac{0.693}{7.8} \times -1\right) = 24.04 \ \mu g/ml$$

Volume of distribution (Vd) is given by

Vd = Body drug content / Plasma drug content = 600 / 24.04 = 24.96 l

---

PROBLEM 26

Calculate the total body clearance (clearance calculated from plasma level decay) of theophylline in a patient in whom the half-life was 9.6 h and in whom the apparent volume of distribution was 23.85 l.

    a. 1.13 l/h
    b. 1.22 l/h
    c. 1.49 l/h
    d. 1.60 l/h
    e. 1.72 l/h

Answer . . . . $\boxed{\text{e}}$

Clearance (Cl) = Apparent volume of distribution (Vd) × Rate constant of plasma level decay (k_{el})

$$= 23.85 \times \frac{0.693}{9.6} = 1.72 \ l/h$$

PROBLEM 27

Metoprolol has a half-life of 3.2 h and an apparent volume of distribution of 4.2 l/kg. Calculate its systemic clearance (whole body clearance calculated from plasma level decay) in a 50-kg patient.

a. $65.6\,h^{-1}$
b. $45.5\,l/h$
c. $3.0\,l.kg^{-1}.h^{-1}$
d. $45.5\,l.kg^{-1}.h^{-1}$
e. $672\,l.kg^{-1}.h^{-1}$

Answer . . . .$\boxed{b}$

$$Cl = Vd \cdot k_{el} = 4.2 \times 50 \times \frac{0.693}{3.2} = 45.5\,l/h$$

PROBLEM 28

A drug was found to be present in the blood of the carotid artery at 6.3 ml/l and in the blood of the jugular vein at 4.6 μg/ml. The blood flow to the brain was 700 ml/min. Assuming the carotid artery and the jugular vein serve only the brain, calculate the ability of the brain to "clear" or "take up" the drug from blood.

a. 188.9 mg/min
b. 700 ml/min
c. 958.7 ml/min
d. 1190 ml/min
e. 188.9 ml/min

Answer . . . .$\boxed{e}$

This is an uptake, or organ clearance, problem, with the unusual feature that a noneliminating organ is involved. The uptake can be presumed to occur as the result of tissue binding, although it could represent metabolism of the drug in the brain (but then the brain would cease to be a noneliminating organ).

$$\text{Uptake} = \left(\frac{Ca - Cv}{Ca}\right) Q = \left(\frac{6.3 - 4.6}{6.3}\right) 700 = 188.9\,\text{ml/min}$$

PROBLEM 29

A drug is given as a 100-mg oral (swallowed) dose. The dose is absorbed with zero-order kinetics. After 30 minutes, gastric lavage shows that 25 mg remain to be absorbed. What is the rate constant of absorption?

    a. $2.5 \, \text{min}^{-1}$
    b. 75 mg/h
    c. $150 \, \text{h}^{-1}$
    d. 2.5 mg/min
    e. 3.3 mg/min

Answer . . . .$\boxed{d}$

Since the absorption shows zero-order kinetics, it occurs at a constant rate and the rate constant of absorption is equal to the rate of absorption. The slope of a graph of amount remaining to be absorbed against time is the rate constant.

$$\text{Slope} = \frac{100 - 25}{0.5} = 150 \, \text{mg/h} = 2.5 \, \text{mg/min}$$

PROBLEM 30

Tetracycline is absorbed from the gastrointestinal tract with first-order kinetics. What was the absorption half-life in a patient in whom 175 mg from an original 250-mg dose was still present in the gastrointestinal tract one hour after the dose?

    a. 2.22 h
    b. 1.94 h
    c. 1.61 h
    d. 1.40 h
    e. 1.05 h

Answer . . . .$\boxed{b}$

The relevant expression for quantity of drug remaining (Qd) as a function of time is

$$Qd_t = Qd_0 \exp(-k_{el} t)$$

In this case

$$175 = 250 \exp(-k_{el} \cdot 1)$$

Taking logarithms,

$$5.16479 = 5.52146 - k_{el}$$

$$\therefore \quad k_{el} = 0.357$$

$$T_{1/2} = 0.693 / k_{el} = 1.94 \, \text{h}$$

PROBLEM 31

A drug is given as a 75 mg oral (swallowed) dose. The dose is absorbed with Michaelis–Menten kinetics. Plasma level measurements indicate that 40 minutes after the dose was administered the instantaneous rate of absorption is 1 mg/min and 25 mg have been absorbed. The K_m for absorption is 25 in the same units as those for the dose dissolved in the lumen of the gastrointestinal tract. Calculate V_{max}.

    a. 10 mg/min
    b. 1.5 mg/min
    c. 1.5 mg.min^{-1}.ml^{-1}
    d. 0.67 mg/min
    e. 0.15 mg/h

Answer . . . .ⓑ

The Michaelis–Menten equation can be recast to relate to disappearance from a site of absorption as follows:

$$\text{Rate of absorption} = \frac{V_{max} \times \text{Amount unabsorbed}}{K_m + \text{Amount unabsorbed}}$$

Thus:

$$V_{max} = \frac{\text{Rate of absorption} \, (K_m + \text{Amount unabsorbed})}{\text{Amount unabsorbed}}$$

In this case:

$$V_{max} = \frac{1[25 + (75 - 25)]}{75 - 25} = \frac{75}{50} = 1.5 \, mg/min$$

PROBLEM 32

Acetaminophen shows saturable (Michaelis–Menten) absorption kinetics. A patient takes a 1 g dose and plasma levels indicate that at the 0.5 h point after dosing the instantaneous rate of absorption is 6 mg/min and 250 mg have been absorbed. The K_m for absorption is 400 in the same units as those for the dose dissolved in the lumen of the gastrointestinal tract. Calculate V_{max}.

    a. 6.0 mg/min
    b. 6.8 mg/min
    c. 7.6 mg/min
    d. 8.4 mg/min
    e. 9.2 mg/min

Answer . . . .$\boxed{e}$

As in the previous question:

$$\text{Rate of absorption} = \frac{V_{max} \times \text{Amount unabsorbed}}{K_m + \text{Amount unabsorbed}}$$

$$6 = \frac{V_{max} \times 750}{400 + 750}$$

$$V_{max} = \frac{6(400 + 750)}{750}$$

$$= 9.2 \, mg/min$$

PROBLEM 33

Calculate k_a, the absorption rate constant, for a drug using the following information: dose, 10 mg; $T_{1/2}$ (of plasma level decay in terminal phase), 13.86 h; apparent volume of distribution, 100 l; Cp_t, when $t = 4$ h, 0.0652 mg/l. Assume $k_a - k_{el} = k_a$ and $F = 1$.

a. $0.28\,h^{-1}$
b. $0.39\,h^{-1}$
c. $0.67\,h^{-1}$
d. $0.56\,h^{-1}$
e. $0.45\,h^{-1}$

Answer . . . .$\boxed{e}$

This is an exercise in using the equation

$$Cp_t = Cp_0[\exp(-k_{el}t) - \exp(-k_a t)]$$

when k_a is unknown. Thus

$$0.0652 = \frac{1 \times 10}{100}\left[\exp\left(-\frac{0.693 \times 4}{13.86}\right) - \exp(-k_a \times 4)\right]$$

$$\exp(-k_a \times 4) = \exp(-0.2) - \frac{0.652}{0.1}$$

$$= 0.8187 - 0.6520$$

$$= 0.1667$$

$$-k_a \times 4 = \ln 0.1667$$

$$= -1.79$$

$$k_a = \frac{1.79}{4}$$

$$= 0.45$$

PROBLEM 34

Lidocaine has a total body clearance of 9.2 ml/kg/minute. What zero-order infusion rate would be needed to induce a steady-state concentration of 10 μg/ml?

a. 92 μg.kg^{-1}.min^{-1}
b. 0.00109 mg.kg^{-1}.min^{-1}

   c. 92 μg/h
   d. 19.2 μg.kg^{-1}.min^{-1}
   e. 8.2 mg/h

Answer . . .   . $\boxed{a}$

With zero-order infusion, the steady-state concentration (Cp$_{ss}$) is given by

$$Cp_{ss} = \text{Input rate } (k_0) / \text{Clearance (Cl)}$$

In this case

$$10 = k_0/9.2$$

$$k_0 = 10 \times 9.2 = 92 \ \mu\text{g.kg}^{-1}.\text{min}^{-1}$$

PROBLEM 35

If a drug has a total body clearance calculated from plasma level decay of 0.5 l/h and is administered at a rate of 50 mg three times a day, the mean steady-state concentration of the drug in plasma, if the drug is administered for a long time, will be (assuming $F = 1$):

   a. 4.2 μg/ml
   b. 12.5 μg/ml
   c. 7200 μg/ml
   d. 1.25 μg/ml
   e. 8.4 μg/ml

Answer . . .   .   /   .   .   .   .   .   . $\boxed{b}$

$$Cp_{ss} = \frac{k_0}{\text{Clearance}} = \frac{150}{0.5 \times 24} = 12.5 \text{ mg/l} = 12.5 \ \mu\text{g/ml}$$

PROBLEM 36

In a patient given Theo-Dur (controlled-release theophylline which leads to minimal fluctuations in theophylline concentration), a single-point measurement of theophylline concentration gave a reading of 10 μg/ml. The daily dose was 500 mg, and the patient had received this dose without change since introduction of therapy six weeks earlier. In this patient, $F = 0.5$ for theophylline and Vd = 35 l. What is the theophylline half-life in this patient?

    a. 21.2 h
    b. 23.3 h
    c. 25.6 h
    d. 27.1 h
    e. 30.0 h

Answer . . . .$\boxed{\text{b}}$

The 24-h area under the curve at steady state was $10 \times 24 = 240$ $\mu g \cdot h$/ml. This equals the area under the curve for a single dose of 500 mg. This can be related to the half-life by means of the clearance (Cl) formula:

$$Cl = Vd \cdot k_{el} = Vd \times 0.693 / T_{1/2}$$

Also

$$Cl = Dose / Area$$

In this case

$$\frac{0.5 \times 500}{240} = 35 \times 0.693 / T_{1/2}$$

$$T_{1/2} = \frac{35 \times 0.693 \times 240}{0.5 \times 500} = 23.3 \text{ h}$$

PROBLEM 37

When the area under the curve from a single dose of a drug is 30 $\mu g \cdot h$/ml, giving the same dose every 0.5 days will result in a mean steady-state concentration of:

    a. 0.4 μg/ml
    b. 360 μg/ml

    c. 2.5 μg/ml
    d. 60 μg/ml
    e. 30 μg/ml

Answer . . . . $\boxed{c}$

$$\text{Area} = 30 \ \mu g \cdot h/ml$$

$$Cp_{ss} = \frac{\text{Area}}{\tau}$$

where τ is the dosing interval. Thus:

$$Cp_{ss} = \frac{30}{0.5 \times 24} = 2.5 \ \mu g/ml$$

PROBLEM 38

A 70 kg patient was receiving 300 mg procaine amide every six hours. His mean Cp_{ss} was 5 μg/ml. What was the half-life of procaine amide in this patient, in whom the drug has an apparent Vd of 1.9 l/kg?

    a. 10.3 h
    b. 9.2 h
    c. 8.1 h
    d. 7.0 h
    e. 5.9 h

Answer . . . . $\boxed{b}$

$$AUC_{ss} = Cp_{ss.mean} \times \tau = 5 \times 6 = 30 \ \mu g \cdot h/ml$$

$$AUC_{ss} = AUC_{first \ dose}$$

$$Cl = Dose/AUC$$

$$Vd \cdot k_{el} = Dose/AUC$$

$$70 \times 1.9 \times \frac{0.693}{T_{1/2}} = 300/30$$

$$T_{1/2} = \frac{70 \times 1.9 \times 0.693 \times 30}{300} = 9.2 \ h$$

PROBLEM 39

Fluphenazine is released in a patient from intramuscular depots at 1 mg/day. It has a steady-state plasma concentration of 1 ng/ml. Its apparent volume of distribution is 10 l/kg. What is its half-life in a 70-kg person?

    a. 0.16 h
    b. 1164 h
    c. 11.64 h
    d. 0.48 h
    e. 0.10 h

Answer . . . .$\boxed{c}$

This is a simple application of the steady-state concept to intramuscular delivery of drugs:

$$Cp_{ss} = k_0 / Vd \cdot k_{el}$$

$$1 \times \frac{1}{1000} = \frac{1}{24 \times 70 \times 10} \times \frac{0.693}{T_{1/2}}$$

$$T_{1/2} = 11.64 \text{ h}$$

PROBLEM 40

If a drug has a half-life of 6 h and it is administered every 24 h, the fluctuation between peak and trough levels at the pseudo-steady state is described adequately by the phrase:

    a. 16-fold increases followed by 100% decrease
    b. 1600% increases followed by 50% decreases
    c. 800% increases followed by 93.75% decreases
    d. 16-fold increases followed by 93.75% decreases
    e. 800% increases followed by 87.5% decreases

Answer . . . .$\boxed{d}$

The dosage interval is $4 \times T_{1/2}$, which means that the fall from peak to trough has to be 93.75%, since the drug concentration declines 50% in one half-life, 75% in two, 87.5% in three, and 93.75% in four. The decision is then between (c) and (d). The increase from trough to peak must restore the earlier peak. This requires multiplication of the trough by:

$$\frac{100}{100 - 93.75} = 16$$

PROBLEM 41

Tolbutamide has a low Vd (apparent volume of distribution), low E (extraction ratio), and low free fraction (α) in plasma. Calculate its intrinsic clearance for the free fraction (Cl_i') given the following information for one particular patient: free fraction, 0.068; Cl_s (systematic clearance—total body clearance from plasma level decay), 18 ml.kg^{-1}.h^{-1}; percent excreted unchanged in urine, 10.

    a. 264.71 ml.kg^{-1}.h^{-1}
    b. 291.18 ml.kg^{-1}.h^{-1}
    c. 238.24 ml.kg^{-1}.h^{-1}
    d. 26.48 ml.kg^{-1}.h^{-1}
    e. 100.00 ml.kg^{-1}.h^{-1}

Answer . . . . $\boxed{c}$

Clearances are additive, so that total clearance is the sum of hepatic and other clearances. In this case:

$$\text{Hepatic clearance } (Cl_H) = \frac{100 - 10}{100} \times Cl_s = 0.9 \times 18 = 16.2 \text{ ml.kg}^{-1}\text{h}^{-1}$$

Because E is low, $Cl_H = Cl_i$.

$$Cl_i = \alpha Cl_i'$$

$$Cl_i' = Cl_i/\alpha = 16.2/0.068 = 238.24 \text{ ml.kg}^{-1}.\text{h}^{-1}$$

PROBLEM 42

In a scientific paper, it was reported that the relative clearance (clearance for an oral dose/clearance for an i.v. dose) for propranolol is 1.82. However, the data showed that the half-life, administered dose, and volume of distribution figures for the two routes of administration were identical. Calculate the extraction ratio of propranolol.

    a. 0
    b. 0.45
    c. 0.50
    d. 0.55
    e. 1

Answer . . . .$\boxed{\text{b}}$

$$\text{Clearance} = \text{Dose}/\text{AUC}$$

where AUC is area under the curve of plasma level against time. Since the Vd, k_{el}, and $T_{1/2}$ values were the same, the clearances were the same. The doses were the same, so the areas after the two doses must have been different, with AUC (oral) less than AUC (i.v.). They could only have been in the ratio $1/1.82 = 0.55$. Thus the extraction ratio (E) is given by:

$$E = 1 - \frac{0.55}{1} = 0.45$$

PROBLEM 43

Calculate the extraction ratio of warfarin in a patient, given the following information: liver blood flow, 1500 ml/min; half-life, 24 h; Vd, 0.2 l/kg; no non-hepatic elimination; weight, 70 kg.

    a. 3.85×10^{-6}
    b. 4.47×10^{-5}
    c. 5.22×10^{-4}

   d. 4.47×10^{-3}
   e. 7.88×10^{-2}

Answer . . . .$\boxed{d}$

Given the characteristics of warfarin:

Hepatic clearance (Cl_H) = Intrinsic clearance (Cl_i)

$\qquad\qquad\qquad$ = Systematic clearance (Cl_s)

$$= Vd \cdot k_{el} = 0.2 \times \frac{0.693}{24} \ 1/kg/h$$

Extraction ratio $(E) = \dfrac{Cl_i}{\text{Liver blood flow } (Q_H) + Cl_i}$

$$= \frac{0.2 \times 0.693/24}{\left(\dfrac{1}{1000} \times \dfrac{1500}{70} \times \dfrac{60}{1}\right) + (0.2 \times 0.693/24)}$$

$$= 4.47 \times 10^{-3}$$

PROBLEM 44

Prednisolone has a normal mean half-life of 3.0 h and a mean volume of distribution of 0.48 1/kg. Calculate the extraction ratio in a 70-kg patient in whom liver blood flow was 1600 ml/min. Urinary excretion is zero.

   a. 0.081
   b. 0.0012
   c. 4.85
   d. 0.000,081
   e. 0.162

Answer . . . .$\boxed{a}$

$$Cl = Q \cdot E$$

where Q is the blood flow and E is the extraction ratio. Thus

$$Vd \cdot k_{el} = Q \cdot E$$

$$\frac{0.693}{3.0} \times 70 \times 0.48 = \frac{60 \times 1600}{1000} \times E$$

$$E = 0.0809$$

PROBLEM 45

Calculate the total intrinsic clearance of a drug, within the liver, when the hepatic extraction ratio is 0.5 in a person in whom the liver blood flow is 1500 ml/min. "Total" drug in this context indicates bound plus nonbound.

    a. 375 ml/h
    b. 750 ml/min
    c. 1500 ml/min
    d. 375 ml/min
    e. 151 l/min

Answer . . . . $\boxed{c}$

$$E = \frac{Cl_i}{Q + Cl_I}$$

$$0.5 = \frac{Cl_i}{1500 + Cl_i}$$

$$Cl_i = (0.5 \times 1500) + (0.5 \times Cl_i) = 1500 \text{ ml/min}$$

PROBLEM 46

---

d-Tubocurarine is eliminated as unchanged drug in urine (40%) and by metabolism in the liver (60%). The mean clearance (total body clearance calculated from plasma level decay) is 2.3 ml/min/kg. What is the mean hepatic clearance?

a. $0.92 \, \text{ml.h}^{-1}.\text{kg}^{-1}$
b. $1.38 \, \text{l.min}^{-1}.\text{kg}^{-1}$
c. $0.92 \, \text{l.h}^{-1}.\text{kg}^{-1}$
d. $1.38 \, \text{ml.h}^{-1}.\text{kg}^{-1}$
e. $1.38 \, \text{ml.min}^{-1}.\text{kg}^{-1}$

Answer . . . . $\boxed{\text{e}}$

Clearances are additive, so

$$Cl_s = Cl_R + Cl_H$$
$$2.3 = (0.4 \times 2.3) + (0.6 \times 2.3)$$
$$Cl_H = 1.38 \, \text{ml.min}^{-1}.\text{kg}^{-1}$$

PROBLEM 47

Phenylbutazone has a low Vd, a low E, and a low free fraction in plasma. Calculate the intrinsic clearance for the free fraction (Cl_i) given the following information: free fraction, 0.039; Cl_s (systemic clearance—total body clearance from plasma level decay), 0.00119 l/kg/h; percent excreted unchanged in urine, zero.

a. $0.067 \, \text{ml.min}^{-1}.\text{kg}^{-1}$
b. $0.00119 \, \text{ml.min}^{-1}.\text{kg}^{-1}$
c. $1.19 \, \text{ml.min}^{-1}\text{kg}^{-1}$
d. $0.51 \, \text{ml.min}^{-1}\text{kg}^{-1}$
e. $0.0199 \, \text{ml.min}^{-1}\text{kg}^{-1}$

Answer . . . . $\boxed{\text{d}}$

In such a case,

$$Cl_H = Cl_s = Cl_i$$

and

$$Cl_s = \alpha Cl_i$$

or

$$Cl_i = \frac{Cl_s}{\alpha} = \frac{0.00119}{0.039} = 0.0305 \, l.kg^{-1}h^{-1} = 30.5 \, ml.kg^{-1}h^{-1}$$
$$= 0.51 \, ml.min^{-1}.kg^{-1}$$

PROBLEM 48

Calculate the extraction ratio of phenybutazone in a 70 kg patient, given the following information: liver blood flow, 1500 ml/min; half-life, 50 h; Vd 0.1 l/kg; no non-hepatic elimination.

     a. 6.46×10^{-5}
     b. 8.88×10^{-6}
     c. 7.92×10^{-6}
     d. 7.22×10^{-6}
     e. 1.08×10^{-3}

Answer . . . .$\boxed{e}$

Note that:

$$E = \frac{Cl_i}{Q_H + Cl_i}$$

In this case:

$$Cl_i = Cl_s = Cl_H$$

$$Cl = Vd \times \frac{0.693}{T_{1/2}} = 0.1 \times 70 \times \frac{0.693}{50} = 0.097 \, l/h = 1.617 \, ml/min$$

Then:

$$E = \frac{1.617}{1500 + 1.617} = 1.08 \times 10^{-3}$$

PROBLEM 49

A drug has an apparent volume of distribution of 1 l/kg and a desired steady-state concentration of 20 μg/ml. What loading dose would be required to achieve this steady state immediately if F (the fraction of the dose reaching the general circulation) is 0.85?

    a. 17.0 mg/kg
    b. 20.0 mg
    c. 23.5 mg
    d. 23.5 mg/kg
    e. 20 mg/kg

Answer . . . .☐d

$$\text{Loading dose} = Cp_{ss} \times Vd \times \frac{1}{F} = 20 \times 1 \times \frac{1}{0.85} = 23.5 \text{ mg/kg}$$

PROBLEM 50

A patient received an intravenous infusion of theophylline (as aminophylline), at 1 mg/min (of theophylline). His weight was 50 kg. The apparent volume of distribution of the theophylline was 0.5 l/kg, the half-life of theophylline was 8 h, and the infusion continued to steady state. Calculate Cp_{ss}.

    a. 24.4 μg/ml
    b. 25.5 μg/ml
    c. 26.4 μg/ml
    d. 27.7 μg/ml
    e. 28.8 μg/ml

Answer . . . .☐d

$$Cp_{ss} = \frac{k_0}{Vd \cdot k_{el}} = \frac{1 \times 60}{50 \times 0.5 \times \dfrac{0.693}{8}} = 27.7 \ \mu\text{g/ml}$$

PROBLEM 51

Ten minutes after completion of a slow intravenous injection of theophylline (as aminophylline) the plasma concentration of theophylline in a 62-kg patient was 22 μg/ml. Given that the half-life of theophylline was 7.8 h in the patient, what was the concentration 40 minutes after completion of the infusion?

    a. 20.9 μg/ml
    b. 21.0 μg/ml
    c. 21.8 μg/ml
    d. 1.5 μg/ml
    e. 0.21 μg/ml

Answer . . . .$\boxed{\text{b}}$

This question requires a knowledge of first-order decay kinetics within a single compartment. The equation required is

$$Cp_t = Cp_0 \exp(-k_{el}t)$$

where Cp_t is the concentration at the second time point and Cp_0 is the concentration at the first time point. Thus

$$Cp_t = 22 \exp\left(-\frac{0.693}{7.8 \times 6.0} \times 30\right) = 21.0 \ \mu g/ml$$

Note that time is expressed with different units in the different pieces of information.

PROBLEM 52

At the end of the infusion in the last question the theophylline body content was 600 mg. The plasma level was calculated to be 22.2 μg/ml. What was the apparent volume of distribution of theophylline?

    a. 0.36 l/kg
    b. 0.39 l/kg
    c. 0.44 l/kg
    d. 0.50 l/kg
    e. 0.60 l/kg

Answer . . . .$\boxed{\text{c}}$

At any time t, the apparent volume of distribution (Vd) is obtained by dividing the amount of the drug in the body at time $t(A_t)$ by the concentration of the drug in plasma at time $t(Cp_t)$. Thus

$$Vd = \frac{A_t}{Cp_t} = \frac{600 \times 1000}{22.2} \times \frac{1}{62} \times \frac{1}{1000} = 0.44 \, 1/kg$$

Note that units must be normalized and that the possible answers do not include 0.44 l/kg multiplied by 62 or 27.28 l. Using the appropriate units, 27.28 l would be a correct answer to the calculation.

PROBLEM 53

In a patient in whom 0.5 l/kg is the correct answer to the previous question and in whom the half-life is 9.0 h, the clearance (whole body clearance calculated from plasma level decay) of theophylline is:

    a. $0.64 \, 1.kg^{-1}.h^{-1}$
    b. $0.0385 \, ml.kg^{-1}.h^{-1}$
    c. $3.85 \, ml.kg^{-1}.h^{-1}$
    d. $0.064 \, ml.kg^{-1}.h^{-1}$
    e. $0.0385 \, 1.kg^{-1}.h^{-1}$

Answer . . . . $\boxed{e}$

Total body clearance, or clearance obtained from plasma level decay when the body behaves as a single compartment, is given by

$$Cl = Vd \cdot k_{el} = 0.5 \times \frac{0.693}{9} = 0.0385 \, 1.kg^{-1}h^{-1}.$$

PROBLEM 54

If theophylline is administered (as aminophylline) by i.v. infusion at 10 mg/min (of theophylline) into a 55-kg person in whom the volume of distribution of theophylline is 0.5 l/kg and in whom the

$T_{1/2}$ of theophylline is 10 h, the concentration in plasma at 20 minutes into the infusion will be:

    a. 7.24 μg/ml
    b. 0.51 μg/ml
    c. 0 μg/ml
    d. 236.1 μg/ml
    e. 1.60 μg/ml

Answer . . . .$\boxed{\text{a}}$

The equation required is

$$Cp_t = \frac{k_0}{Vd \cdot k_{el}} [1 - \exp(-k_{el}t)]$$

where k_0 is the rate of zero-order infusion. Thus

$$Cp_t = \frac{10 \times 60}{0.5 \times 55 \times \dfrac{0.693}{10}} \left[1 - \exp\left(-\frac{0.693}{10 \times 60} \times 20\right)\right] = 7.24 \ \mu g/ml$$

Note the need to normalize the units of time. Also, because calculators "round off" numbers, it is best to use a floating decimal point and "round off" only at the end. Alternatively, if your answer is slightly different from 7.24, but not similar to any of the others, work the stages of the calculation in a different order and compare possible answers.

PROBLEM 55

In the patient in the last question, given an infusion of 1 mg/min continued indefinitely, what will be the steady-state concentration?

    a. 17,325 μg/ml
    b. 5.25 μg/ml
    c. 315 μg/ml
    d. 31.48 μg/ml
    e. 34,650 μg/ml

Answer . . . .$\boxed{\text{d}}$

At steady state

$$Cp_t = \frac{k_0}{Vd \cdot k_{el}} = \frac{1 \times 60}{0.5 \times 55 \times \dfrac{0.693}{10}} = 31.48 \ \mu g/ml$$

Note the warnings in the previous example.

PROBLEM 56

Eight percent of the body content of theophylline is excreted unchanged in urine. In a patient in whom the half-life is 7.5 h, the rate constant for renal excretion is:

a. $0.00739 \ min^{-1}$
b. $0.00739 \ h^{-1}$
c. $0.4435 \ min^{-1}$
d. $4.435 \ h^{-1}$
e. $0.01478 \ h^{-1}$

Answer . . . . .b

Rate constants are additive, so

$$k_{el} = k_m + k_e$$

where k_m is the first-order rate constant for metabolism and k_e is the first-order rate constant for excretion of the unchanged drug. Thus

$$\frac{0.693}{7.5} = \left(0.92 \times \frac{0.693}{7.5}\right) + \left(0.08 \times \frac{0.693}{7.5}\right)$$

As a component of this

$$k_e = 0.08 \times \frac{0.693}{7.5} = 0.00739 \ h^{-1}$$

PROBLEM 57

Procaine amide has an apparent volume of distribution of 1.9 ± 0.3 (mean $\pm$ S.E.M.) l/kg. This probably indicates distribution through a two-compartment system. However, distribution is rapid and for most purposes the body can be considered as behaving as a single homogeneous procaine amide compartment. Assume this to apply in a patient aged 45, weighing 71 kg, who received a 100-mg i.v. dose. The half-life in this patient was previously determined to be 4.5 h. Using the mean value for Vd, calculated Cp_t where $= 5$ min.

    a. 0.4630 μg/ml
    b. 0.7413 μg/ml
    c. 0.7508 μg/ml
    d. 0.7319 μg/ml
    e. 0.3432 μg/ml

Answer . . . .$\boxed{d}$

Use the equations:

$$Cp_t = Cp_0 \exp(-k_{el}t)$$
$$Vd = Dose/Cp_0$$

Then

$$Cp_t = \frac{100}{1.9 \times 71} \exp\left(\frac{-0.693}{4.5} \times \frac{5}{60}\right)$$
$$= 0.7319 \ \mu g/ml$$

PROBLEM 58

It is considered that 5 μg/ml of procaine amide is the minimum for useful clinical effect. However, procaine amide cannot be given as a single i.v. dose of sufficient magnitude to immediately induce 5 μg/ml because dangerous hypotension would result. It can be given by intermittent i.v. bolus doses of 100 mg repeated at 5 min intervals. In a patient in whom the correct answer in the previous question was 0.7319 μg/ml, how many i.v. injections would be needed such that 5 μg/ml (at least) was present at the end of the last 5-min dosage interval?

    a. 5   c. 7   e. 9
    b. 6   d. 8

Answer . . . .$\boxed{d}$

PROBLEM 58

Illustration

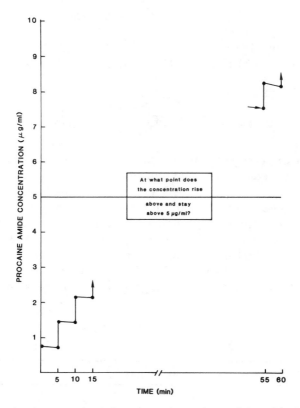

Fig. 14. Sketch of progression of concentrations of procaine amide implicit in Problem 58.

This requires repeated use of the equations used in the previous problem. Also, it is useful to draw a sketch to represent the situation being studied (see Fig. 14). The first dose (previous question) induced a peak (0 time) concentration of

$$Cp_0 = 100/(1.9 \times 71) = 0.74 \ \mu g/ml$$

and a trough (5 min, calculated) of 0.73 $\mu g/ml$. The second dose added 0.74 to 0.73 to give 1.47. Treating this as a new Cp_0 in the equation

$$Cp_t = Cp_0 \exp\left(\frac{-0.693}{4.5} \times \frac{5}{60}\right)$$

in which Cp_t is now the trough at 10 minutes on the graph, but in which t still equals 5 min (5 min after the most recent dose), the second trough is found to be 1.45 $\mu g/ml$. Similarly, the third peak value is 2.19 $\mu g/ml$. The question asks how many 5-min intervals will pass before the trough equals or exceeds 5 $\mu g/ml$. The fourth, fifth, sixth, seventh, and eighth troughs will be 2.85, 3.53, 4.21, 4.88, and 5.54, so that the answer to the question is 8. Note that $Cp_0 \times 7 = 0.74 \times 7 = 5.18$, which fails to allow for the (albeit small) important falls from peak to trough in each dosage interval.

PROBLEM 59

Procaine amide has an apparent mean volume of distribution (Vd) of 1.9 l/kg and distribution is effectively through a one-compartment system. The half-life of procaine amide in the patient in the previous question was known to be 4.5 h. What total dose would be needed by constant-rate infusion at 20 mg/min to induce a plasma concentration of 5 $\mu g/ml$?

    a. 1.00 mg
    b. 5.00 mg
    c. 11.76 mg
    d. 655.0 mg
    e. 705.6 mg

Answer . . . . $\boxed{e}$

This problem focuses attention on infusion to steady state but asks for the *cumulative* amount administered when a certain concentration is reached. The equation is

$$Cp_t = \frac{k_0}{Vd \cdot k_{el}} [1 - \exp(-k_{el}t)]$$

in which t is unknown and Cp_t is 5 $\mu g/ml$. Once t is calculated, it can be multiplied by the infusion rate to give the cumulative dose:

$$5 = \frac{20,000}{1.9 \times 1000 \times 71 \times \dfrac{0.693}{4.5 \times 60}} \left[1 - \exp\left(\frac{-0.693}{4.5 \times 60}\right)t\right]$$

for which $t = 35.28$ min (or 0.588 h). Using this, dose $= 35.28 \times 20 = 705.6$ mg.

PROBLEM 60

In the previous question, having induced 5 $\mu g/ml$, what infusion rate would then be needed to *maintain* 5 $\mu g/ml$?

    a. 1.73 mg/min
    b. 2.00 mg/min
    c. 106 mg/h
    d. 1.5 mg/min
    e. 1.73 mg/h

Answer . . . . $\boxed{a}$

The infusion in the previous question did not continue to steady state (which would have been achieved after 3–5 times the half-life had elapsed, or 13.5–22.5 hours, and which would have involved a Cp_{ss} in the lethal range). This question tells us to treat 5 $\mu g/ml$ as a desirable Cp_{ss}. At steady state

$$\text{Infusion rate} = \text{Clearance} \times \text{Concentration} = 1.9 \times 71 \times \frac{0.693}{4.5} \times 5$$

$$= 103.9 \text{ mg/h} = 1.73 \text{ mg/min}$$

PROBLEM 61

As stated before, procaine amide has an apparent mean volume of distribution (Vd) of 1.9 l/kg. Distribution is effectively through a one-compartment system. The half-life of procaine amide in our patient is known to be 4.5 h. Using these constants, what oral dose would be needed to achieve 5 μg/ml six hours after its administration, assuming that the fraction of the dose reaching the general circulation is 0.83 at all dose levels and that absorption of this fraction occurs with first-order kinetics and is 90% complete in one hour?

    a. 1000 mg/kg
    b. 1915 mg
    c. 2.5 g
    d. 20 mg/kg
    e. 1915 g

Answer . . . . .b

The core equation for this problem is

$$Cp_t = \frac{F \cdot D}{Vd} \cdot \left(\frac{k_a}{k_a - k_{el}} \right) \cdot [\exp(-k_{el}t) - \exp(-k_a t)]$$

in which D is the unknown. However, we do not have a value for k_a, but this is obtainable from

$$Qd_t = Qd_0 \exp(-k_a t)$$

in which Qd_t is the quantity *unabsorbed* at time t and Qd_0 is the quantity unabsorbed at time 0. We actually only need the ratio Qd_t/Qd_0, for obvious reasons. In the present case,

$$\frac{1 - 0.9}{1} = \exp(-k_a \times 1)$$

Solving for k_a,

$$k_a = 2.3 \, h^{-1}$$

Then,

$$5 = \frac{0.83 \times D}{1.9 \times 71} \left(\frac{2.3}{2.3 - \frac{0.693}{4.5}} \right) \left[\exp\left(\frac{-0.693}{4.5} \cdot 6 \right) - \exp(-2.3 \times 6) \right]$$

$$= 6.15 \times 10^{-3} \times D \times 1.07(0.396928 - 1.0156 \times 10^{-6})$$

$$D = \frac{5 \times 10^3}{6.15 \times 1.07 \times 0.39690}$$

$$= 1915 \, mg$$

PROBLEM 62

Noting that procaine amide has an apparent mean volume of distribution (Vd) of 1.9 l/kg and that distribution is effectively through a one-compartment system, calculate the systematic clearance (clearance calculated from plasma level decay) of procaine amide in the patient with a 4.5-h half-life for procaine amide.

    a. 0.2926 l/h
    b. 29.26 ml.kg^{-1}.h^{-1}
    c. 20.77 l.kg^{-1}.h^{-1}
    d. 207.7 l/h
    e. 0.2926 l.kg^{-1}h^{-1}

Answer . . . .$\boxed{e}$

$$Cl = Vd \cdot k_{el} = 1.9 \times \frac{0.693}{4.5} = 0.2926 \, l.kg^{-1}.h^{-1}$$

PROBLEM 63

The following is the equation for the plasma concentration of diazepam given intravenously to a certain patient:

$$Cp_t = 3.45 \exp(-2.97\,t) + 1.65 \exp(-0.21\,t)$$

The dose was 10 mg/kg. Calculate Area $(0\to\infty)$; concentrations are in ng/ml and t is in hours.

    a. 4.98 ng·h/ml
    b. 5.99 ng·h/ml
    c. 7.00 ng·h/ml
    d. 8.01 ng·h/ml
    e. 9.02 ng·h/ml

Answer . . . . .e

The following equation fits the general model for a two-compartment case:

$$Cp_t = A \exp(-\alpha t) + B \exp(-\beta t)$$

From this, area under the curve (AUC) is given by:

$$\mathrm{AUC} = \frac{A}{\alpha} + \frac{B}{\beta} = \frac{3.45}{2.97} + \frac{1.65}{0.21} = 9.02 \text{ ng·h/ml}$$

PROBLEM 64

Calculate the clearance from the central compartment for a patient in whom the correct answer in the previous question was 7 ng·h/ml.

    a. $70\,\mathrm{l.kg^{-1}.h^{-1}}$
    b. $1428.6\,\mathrm{l.kg^{-1}.h^{-1}}$
    c. $1.4286\,\mathrm{l.kg^{-1}.h^{-1}}$
    d. $70{,}000\,\mathrm{l.kg^{-1}.h^{-1}}$
    e. $7.143\,\mathrm{l.kg^{-1}.h^{-1}}$

Answer . . . . .b

Regardless of the number of compartments, clearance (Cl) from the central compartment is given by

$$Cl = Dose/AUC$$

It can be shown that this is equal to $k_{10}Vc$ where k_{10} is given by

$$k_{10} = \frac{A + B}{A/\alpha + B/\beta}$$

and Vc is the volume of the central compartment.
In this case:

$$k_{10}Vc = \frac{10 \times 1000}{7} = 1428.6 \, \text{l.kg}^{-1}.\text{h}^{-1}$$

The rate constant k_{10} is that of elimination from the central compartment. Note that k_{10} is greater than β.

PROBLEM 65

Calculate the renal clearance of sulfamethazine, given the following information: midpoint plasma level, 26 μg/ml; time of urine collection, 20 min; urine volume collected, 15 ml; urine concentration of drug, 350 μg/ml.

    a. 269 ml/min
    b. 121 ml/h
    c. 10.1 ml/min
    d. 303 ml/h
    e. 0.101 l/min

Answer . . . .$\boxed{c}$

$$Cl = \frac{UV}{P} = \frac{350 \times \dfrac{15}{20}}{26} = 10.1 \, \text{ml/min}$$

PROBLEM 66

Meperidine has a mean half-life in plasma of 3.2 h. Given that 20% is excreted unchanged in urine, what is the rate constant of renal excretion?

a. $0.032 \, h^{-1}$
b. $0.043 \, h^{-1}$
c. $0.054 \, h^{-1}$
d. $0.065 \, h^{-1}$
e. $0.076 \, h^{-1}$

Answer . . . . $\boxed{b}$

We can make the assumption that the remaining 80% of elimination is hepatic, as this will not affect the answer. Thus

$$k_{el} = 0.693/3.2 = k_R + k_H$$

$$k_R = 0.2 \times k_{el} = 0.2 \times 0.693/3.2 = 0.0433 \, h^{-1}$$

PROBLEM 67

Estimate the revised minocycline dose to be given to a patient whose dose during normal renal function was 300 mg per day, when 10% of the dose was excreted unchanged in urine. The revised dose was required when renal function fell by 80%.

a. 300 mg
b. 294 mg
c. 270 mg
d. 276 mg
e. 264 mg

Answer . . . . $\boxed{d}$

A correction is needed for only the renally excreted minocycline, which accounts for 10% of the dose. The dose should therefore be reduced by

$$\frac{(100 - 20)}{100} \times \frac{10}{100} \times 300 = 24 \, mg$$

to 276 mg.

PROBLEM 68

A female patient undergoing treatment with an antibiotic was known to have a half-life for the drug of 13.6 h. When placed on dialysis, her dialysis clearance of the drug was 1.76 l/h. The volume of distribution of the drug was 54 l in both circumstances. What was the half-life of the drug during dialysis? Note that dialysis clearance is clearance caused by dialysis.

    a. 8.25 h
    b. 7.75 h
    c. 7.40 h
    d. 7.10 h
    e. 6.75 h

Answer . . . . $\boxed{\text{a}}$

Note that

Clearance on dialysis = endogenous clearance + dialysis clearance

in that *dialysis clearance* is clearance caused by the artificial kidney. This type of problem is best solved with a table:

	Off dialysis	On dialysis
Vd	54 l	54 l
$T_{1/2}$	13.6 h	8.25 h
$k_{el} = \dfrac{0.693}{T_{1/2}}$	0.051 h^{-1}	0.084 h^{-1}
Cl = Vd · k_{el}	2.75 l/h	4.51 l/h

You are given the information on Vd and the $T_{1/2}$ off dialysis. From this, you calculate k_{el} and Cl off dialysis. Dialysis clearance added to endogenous clearance (off dialysis) gives clearance on dialysis:

$$1.76 + 2.75 = 4.51$$

Working back through the table, the $T_{1/2}$ on dialysis emerges as 8.25 h.

PROBLEM 69

An anephric patient on dialysis because of uremia required an antibiotic. The antibiotic had an apparent volume of distribution of 66.3 l. Its plasma half-life during dialysis was 5.7 h. Its clearance from plasma when the patient was off dialysis was 4.77 ml/h. Calculate the proportion of the clearance during the dialysis caused by endogenous clearance.

     a. 39.32%
     b. 41.04%
     c. 49.67%
     d. 57.22%
     e. 59.18%

Answer . . . .$\boxed{e}$

	Off dialysis	On dialysis
Vd (l)	66.3	66.3
$T_{1/2}$ (h)	—	5.7
k_{el} (h^{-1})	—	0.122
Cl (l/h)	4.77	8.06

Dialysis adds $8.06 - 4.77 = 3.29$ l/h or 40.8%.

Endogenous clearance contributed $\dfrac{4.77}{8.06} \times 100 = 59.18\%$.

PROBLEM 70

Chloramphenicol is eliminated almost entirely by metabolism. It is a "low-E" drug. Its half-life in normals is 2.3 h. What would its half-life be in a liver disease patient whose indocyanine green clearance was 50% of normal and in whom all other tests of liver function were normal?

     a. 1.15 h
     b. 2.30 h
     c. 3.45 h
     d. 4.60 h
     e. 5.75 h

Answer . . . . $\boxed{b}$

Low-extraction-ratio ("low-E") drugs are most affected in regard to hepatic clearance by enzyme activity. This contrasts with "high-E" drugs, for which hepatic clearance is most affected by hepatic blood flow. Indocyanine green clearance evaluates hepatic blood flow, which is not a factor in the case in the problem. Thus no change is to be expected if other tests of liver function (e.g., antipyrine half-life) show no change.

PROBLEM 71

In a patient with normal renal function, 65% of digoxin was excreted unchanged, and the plasma half-life of the drug was 1.7 days. The patient then went into partial renal failure and his creatinine clearance dropped from 125 ml/min to 50 ml/min. Calculate the expected half-life in his partially anuric state.

    a. 2.62 days
    b. 2.15 days
    c. 12.16 hours
    d. 3.33 days
    e. 2.79 days

Answer . . . . $\boxed{e}$

The equation required is

$$k_{el(U)} = k_{NR} + \left[k_{R(N)} \times \frac{50}{125} \right]$$

where U indicates uremic, NR indicates non-renal, R indicates renal, and N indicates normal. The value of k_{NR} is equal to $k_{el(U)}$ when creatinine clearance is zero. The calculation uses the fraction excreted unchanged:

$$k_{NR} = 0.35 \times \frac{0.693}{1.7} = 0.1427$$

$$k_{R(N)} = 0.65 \times \frac{0.693}{1.7} = 0.2650$$

$$k_{R(N)} \times \frac{50}{125} = 0.1060$$

$$k_{el(U)} = 0.1427 + 0.1060 = 0.2487$$

$$T_{1/2} = \frac{0.693}{0.2487} = 2.79 \text{ days}$$

PROBLEM 72

A patient on digoxin has both renal and hepatic impairment. In place of the normal creatinine clearance of 125 ml/min, his creatinine clearance was 50 ml/min. His ability to metabolize digoxin was 50% of normal. Digoxin is excreted 63% unchanged. By what proportion was his digoxin half-life different from that of "normals"?

    a. 0.437 lower
    b. 0.563 higher
    c. 0.586 higher
    d. 0.404 lower
    e. 0.586 lower

Answer . . . .$\boxed{b}$

$$k_{el} = k_R + k_{NR}$$

where NR indicates "non-renal."

Normal: $k_{el} = 0.63 \, k_{el} + 0.37 \, k_{el}$

Patient: $k_{el} = \left(\frac{50}{125} \times 0.63 \, k_{el} \right) + (0.5 \times 0.37 \, k_{el})$

Fraction: $\dfrac{k_{el} \text{ (Patient)}}{k_{el} \text{ (Normal)}} = \left(\dfrac{50}{125} \times 0.63 \right) + (0.5 \times 0.37) = 0.252 + 0.185$

$$= 0.437$$

The fractional *reduction* in k_{el}, and therefore fractional *increase* in $T_{1/2}$, was 0.563.

PROBLEM 73

Nadolol is 75% excreted unchanged in urine, has a normal half-life of 16 h, and has a hepatic extraction ratio of 0.3. Calculate its half-life in a patient in whom the normal creatinine clearance of 125 ml/min had dropped to 75 ml/min, in whom the antipyrine half-life was twice normal, and in whom the indocyanine green clearance was half of normal.

    a. 31.94 h
    b. 27.83 h
    c. 23.72 h
    d. 19.84 h
    e. 17.22 h

Answer . . . .$\boxed{b}$

$$k_{el} = k_R + k_{NR}$$

$$\frac{0.693}{16} = \left(0.75 \times \frac{0.693}{16}\right) + \left(0.25 + \frac{0.693}{16}\right)$$

$$k_{el(u)} = \left(0.75 \times \frac{0.693}{16} \times \frac{75}{125}\right) + \left(0.25 \times \frac{0.693}{16} \times 0.5\right) = 0.0249$$

$$T_{1/2} = 27.83 \text{ h}$$

Note that k_R is proportional to creatinine clearance. Also, since the drug has a low hepatic extraction ratio, its hepatic clearance is much influenced by enzyme activity (assessed by means of the antipyrine half-life) and little influenced by liver blood flow (assessed by means of indocyanine green clearance).

PROBLEM 74

Congestive heart failure (CHF) leads to a reduced volume of distribution for lidocaine. If the normal Vd is 1.1 l/kg, and the normal half-life is unchanged at 1.8 h in CHF, what is the clearance if Vd is reduced by 20%?

a. $0.42\,l.kg^{-1}.h^{-1}$
b. $0.38\,l.kg^{-1}.h^{-1}$
c. $0.34\,l.kg^{-1}.h^{-1}$
d. $0.20\,l.kg^{-1}.h^{-1}$
e. $0.15\,l.kg^{-1}.h^{-1}$

Answer . . . .$\boxed{\text{c}}$

$$Cl = Vd \cdot k_{el} = 0.81 \times 1.1 \times \frac{0.693}{1.8} = 0.3388\,l/kg^{-1}/h^{-1}$$

PROBLEM 75

Congestive heart failure (CHF) leads to a reduced volume of distri-bution of lidocaine. If the drug has a normal Vd of $1.1\,kg^{-1}$ and a normal half-life of 1.8 h which is unchanged in CHF, what is the *change* in clearance when CHF reduces the Vd by 10%?

a. Up $0.0423\,l.kg^{-1}.h^{-1}$
b. Up $0.4235\,l.kg^{-1}.h^{-1}$
c. No change
d. Down $0.3812\,l.kg^{-1}.h^{-1}$
e. Down $0.0423\,l.kg^{-1}.h^{-1}$

Answer . . . .$\boxed{\text{e}}$

$$Cl = Vd \times \frac{0.693}{T_{1/2}}$$

Normal: $Cl = 1.1 \times \dfrac{0.693}{1.8} = 0.4235\,l.kg^{-1}.h^{-1}$

CHF: $Cl = 0.9 \times 1.1 \times \dfrac{0.693}{1.8} = 0.3812\,l.kg^{-1}.h^{-1}$

The change is a decrease of $0.0423\,l.kg^{-1}.h^{-1}$

PROBLEM 76

Lidocaine has a normal clearance of $12.2\,ml.min^{-1}.kg^{-1}$. If a patient with congestive heart failure receives the standard infusion of lidocaine, by what factor will the steady-state plasma levels in this patient exceed those of a "normal" control, bearing in mind that the indocyanine green clearance in the patient is $1.7 \, ml.min^{-1}.kg^{-1}$?

    a. 4.14
    b. 5.15
    c. 6.45
    d. 7.17
    e. 8.18

Answer . . . .$\boxed{c}$

Indocyanine green clearance assesses liver blood flow. Since lidocaine clearance is 90% controlled by liver blood flow, we can conclude that the lidocaine clearance in the patient was $100/90 \times 1.7 \, ml.min^{-1}.kg^{-1} = 1.89 \, ml.min^{-1}.kg^{-1}$. Plasma levels are inversely proportional to clearance, so the plasma levels in the patient will be $12.2/1.89 = 6.45$ times those of the normal.

PROBLEM 77

Calculate the percentage acetylation of sulfamethazine in a patient, given the following information: concentration of sulfamethazine in plasma at 5.5 hours post-dosage, 16.0 $\mu g/ml$; concentration of acetylsulfamethazine in plasma at 8 hours post-dosage of sulfamethazine, 51.0 $\mu g/ml$; half-life of exponential decline of sulfamethazine in plasma from 4 to 8 hours post-dosage, 1.566 h. Ignore the molecular weight differences between the two compounds.

    a. 10.4%
    b. 9.4%
    c. 100.0%
    d. 0.0%
    e. 90.6%

Answer . . . .$\boxed{e}$

The percentage of sulfamethazine acetylated in plasma reflects the activity of the drug-acetylating enzymes responsible for metabolism of the sulfonamides, isoniazid, and certain other drugs. Knowledge of acetylator status is useful in guiding isoniazid therapy. In the problem, the concentrations of the two compounds at the same time are needed. Thus, for sulfamethazine:

$$Cp_t = Cp_0 \exp(-k_{el}t) = 16 \exp\left(\frac{-0.693}{1.566} \times 2.5\right) = 5.29$$

$$\%Acetylation = \frac{51.0}{51.0 + 5.29} \times 100 = 90.6\%$$

PROBLEM 78

Calculate a debrisoquine MR (metabolic ratio) number given the following information: concentration of debrisoquine in urine, 22.6 μg/ml; urine volume collected in the 8-h collection period, 322 ml; amount of 4-hydroxydebrisoquine in urine, 6.44 mg.

    a. 0.88
    b. 20.0
    c. 0.14
    d. 1.13
    e. 9.04

Answer . . . .$\boxed{d}$

The MR is a measure of the activity of the P-450 system of the liver. A low ratio indicates a high ability to hydroxylate drugs. A high ratio indicates a low activity. Patients with a high ratio are especially at risk of toxicity from certain drugs, including phenytoin.

$$MR = \frac{\text{Debrisoquine concentration}}{\text{4-Hydroxydebrisoquine concentration}} = \frac{22.6}{6.44 \times 1000/322}$$

$$= 1.13$$

PROBLEM 79

Calculate the dibucaine number in a patient given the following information: benzoylcholine hydrolysis rate in the absence of dibucaine, 0.65 moles/h; benzoylcholine hydrolysis rate in the presence of dibucaine, 0.49 moles/h.

    a. 132.65
    b. 75.4
    c. 32.65
    d. 24.6
    e. 0.25

Answer . . . .$\boxed{d}$

The dibucaine number evaluates plasma pseudocholinesterase activity. Benzoylcholine is used as a substrate for the enzyme in an *in vitro* test. Dibucaine inhibits the metabolism of benzoylcholine. The degree of inhibition is used to evaluate the function of pseudocholinesterase, which is important in controlling the duration of action of succinylcholine.

$$DN = 100 \times \left[1 - \frac{\text{(Hydrolysis rate with dibucaine)}}{\text{(Hydrolysis rate without dibucaine)}} \right]$$

$$= 100 \times \left[1 - \frac{0.49}{0.65} \right] = 24.6$$

PROBLEM 80

Succinylcholine was given intravenously at four dose levels to a healthy volunteer, and the durations of respiratory paralysis induced were:

Dose (mg)	50	100	200	400
Time (min)	5.0	10.2	15.0	19.9

The threshold dose for effect was, therefore,

    a. 50 mg
    b. 50 mg/kg
    c. 1.38 mg
    d. 24 mg
    e. 1.38 mg/kg

Answer . . . .$\boxed{d}$

Two of the answers, (b) and (e), are impossible because the weight of the volunteer is not known. Answer (a) is impossible because 50 mg causes 5.0 min of paralysis. This leaves a decision between 1.38 mg and 24 mg. Instinctively, 24 mg is more likely to be correct. In fact, the data illustrate addition of a *constant increment* for each doubling of the dose, so without drawing a graph, 24 mg is seen to be correct.

PROBLEM 81

Diazepam is 99.4% bound to plasma protein in normal corcumstances. Calculate K, the equilibrium constant of binding, assuming that there is a single population of binding sites, one site per molecule of protein, that the binding protein has a molecular weight of 65,000 and is present at 4% in plasma, and that KPt is *much* greater than 1.

    a. 2.41×10^2
    b. 2.51×10^3
    c. 2.61×10^4
    d. 2.71×10^5
    e. 2.81×10^6

Answer . . . . $\boxed{\text{d}}$

When K and Pt are both high, the free fraction (α) is given by

$$\alpha = 1/nKPt$$

In this case: $\dfrac{100 - 99.4}{100} = 1 \Big/ \left(1 \times K \times 40 \times \dfrac{1}{65,000}\right)$

from which $K = 2.71 \times 10^5$.

PROBLEM 82

Digitoxin is 90% bound to plasma protein in normal circumstances. Calculate K, the equilibrium constant of binding, assuming that there is a single population of binding sites, one site per molecule of protein, that the binding protein has a molecular weight of 65,000 and is present at 4% in plasma, and that KPt is much greater than 1.

    a. 1.212×10^3
    b. 1.625×10^4
    c. 2.736×10^5
    d. 3.840×10^5
    e. 4.500×10^5

Answer . . . . .b

In the circumstances described

$$\alpha = 1/n\text{KPt}$$

$$0.1 = \cfrac{1}{1 \times K \times \cfrac{40}{65{,}000}}$$

$$K = \frac{65{,}000}{0.1 \times 40} = 1.625 \times 10^4 \, \text{M}$$

PROBLEM 83

A patient was found to be suffering from nystagmus attributable to phenytoin therapy. Plasma phenytoin was 32 μg/ml when the dosage was 700 mg/day and then 20.55 μg/ml six weeks later when the dosage was 500 mg/day. After another six weeks, at 300 mg/day, the nystagmus was gone. Calculate the drug concentration in plasma on the 300-mg/day regimen.

    a. 850 μg/ml
    b. 83.8 μg/ml
    c. 26.7 μg/ml
    d. 11.2 μg/ml
    e. 5.5 μg/ml

Answer . . . . .d

Dose	Cp_{ss}	Dose/Cp_{ss}
700	32.00	21.88
500	20.55	24.33
300	x	y

The linear relationship is inverse, with dose proportional to $1/(\text{Dose}/\text{Cp}_{ss})$. The change in $\text{Dose}/\text{Cp}_{ss}$ for a 200-mg dose reduction is 2.45, so $y = 24.33 + 2.45 = 26.78$. If $\text{Dose}/\text{Cp}_{ss} = 26.78$ with dose $= 300$, then Cp_{ss} is equal to 11.2 $\mu g/ml$.

PROBLEM 84

Nitroglycerin has a plasma half-life *in vivo* of 2 min. *In vitro*, in whole blood, its half-life is 6 min. If an *in vivo* inhibitor was introduced and this inhibitor completely prevented only that part of the nitroglycerin elimination uniquely associated with the *in vivo* situation, by what proportion would the clearance decrease *in vivo*?

    a. One-third
    b. A factor of three
    c. 70%
    d. Two-thirds
    e. Zero

Answer . . . .$\boxed{d}$

The half-life *in vivo* is 2 min, for a rate constant of 0.3465 min^{-1}. The half-life in blood *in vitro* is 6 min for a rate constant of 0.1155 min^{-1}. Rate constants, but not half-lives, are additive so

$$\frac{0.3465 - 0.1155}{0.3465} = 0.67$$

for a two-thirds reduction in rate constant. Since rate constants are proportional to clearance, the clearance would decrease by two-thirds.

PROBLEM 85

Calculate the i.v. infusion dose (in mg/min) of succinylcholine required to maintain a body content of 20 mg following a 20-mg i.v. bolus dose in a patient with a succinylcholine half-life of 12 min.

    a. 1.155
    b. 1.266

   c. 1.377
   d. 1.488
   e. 1.599

Answer . . . .$\boxed{a}$

This is an exercise in steady-state kinetics with respect to quantity of drug in the body. At steady state, this quantity is constant and its rate of change is zero. Hence

$$dQd/dt = k_0 - k_{el}Qd = 0$$

The infusion rate, k_0, is the unknown so

$$x = k_{el}Qd = \frac{0.693}{12} \times 20 = 1.155 \, mg/min$$

PROBLEM 86

Calculate the mean residence time (MRT) for a drug with a terminal-phase half-life of 36 hours.

   a. 36.0 h
   b. 51.9 h
   c. 0.19 h^{-1}
   d. 51.9 h^{-1}
   e. 36.0 h^{-1}

Answer . . . .$\boxed{b}$

The MRT for a drug administered by intravenous bolus injection is given by a formula not listed in the introductory section:

$$MRT = 1/\lambda_z$$

where λ_z is the rate constant of decay during the terminal phase. Thus in this case:

$$\lambda_z = 0.693/36 = 0.01925 \, h^{-1}$$

$$MRT = 51.94 \, h$$

MRT measurements are useful because of their additivity and because the MRT can be obtained from the ratio of the first moment area under the curve (AUMC) are the zeroth moment area under the curve (AUC), as well as from terminal-phase rate constant measurements. Thus

$$MRT = AUMC/AUC$$

Because of additivity

$$k_a = MRT_{oral\ dose} - MRT_{i.v.\ dose}$$

PART III:
Single Answer
Factual Questions

PROBLEM 87

In the expression LADME, the capital letter A is the initial letter of

    a. adsorption
    b. area under the curve
    c. availability
    d. accumulation
    e. absorption

Answer ⌊e⌋

The mnemonic LADME is a useful contraction of the initial letters of:

Liberation	release of the drug from its dosage form;
Absorption	transfer of the drug from the site of liberation into the blood stream;
Distribution	transfer of the drug through the fluids and tissues of the body, including binding to sites of action and storage within tissues;
Metabolism	conversion of the drug to active or inactive products to make excretion possible;
Excretion	transfer of the drug out of the body through the kidney and other excretary organs.

Avoid confusion of absorption with adsorption, which refers to the surface interaction of drugs with proteins (reversible plasma protein binding).

PROBLEM 88

In the expression LADME, the capital letter E is the initial letter of

    a. extraction ratio
    b. elimination
    c. excretion
    d. extracellular fluid
    e. enzyme

Answer ⌊c⌋

See the previous question for a full description of the LADME mnemonic. The distinction to be made in this question is between elimination and excretion. Elimination is generally considered to be the sum of metabolism and excretion.

PROBLEM 89

Whole blood but not serum

   a. contains no heparin
   b. contains fibrinogen
   c. always contains citric acid as an anticoagulent
   d. contains albumin
   e. contains potassium

Answer   b

This is intended to focus attention on the need for precision in use of terms. Blood, serum, and plasma are not synonymous—they are three different biological media. In fact, serum is nonphysiological. All three contain heparin. None *always* contain citric acid *as an* anticoagulant. Serum contains albumin and potassium, leaving (b) as the only possible answer.

PROBLEM 90

If a drug is a weak base and its absorption is affected by the pH of gastrointestinal contents, its absorption will be favored by or in

   a. conditions in the stomach more than elsewhere
   b. conditions in the intestine more than elsewhere
   c. areas of relatively low pH
   d. areas of relatively high acidity
   e. gastric acid secretion induced by food

Answer   b

The weak base is relatively insoluble under relatively alkaline aqueous conditions. When the aqueous fluid is unfavorable to solution, the drug diffuses more readily into the lipophilic membranes of the absorbing organ. The intestinal contents are less acidic (pH 5.3–7.0) than the stomach contents, favoring absorption.

PROBLEM 91

The "first-pass effect" of a drug is most likely to be a significant factor affecting the proportion of a dose which reaches the general circulation for drugs which

    a. are highly protein bound
    b. are excreted in bile
    c. are only given by intramuscular injection
    d. have a high hepatic extraction ratio
    e. are eliminated entirely by renal excretion

Answer   ⒟

The first-pass effect is metabolism of drugs during transfer through the gastrointestinal mucosa and muscle, the portal circulation, and the liver. For the first-pass effect to be a significant factor, the enzymes concerned must be capable of a high level of activity, as a large quantity of drug is exposed to them during a short period of time. Thus drugs with a high hepatic extraction ratio are most likely to be subject to a significant first-pass effect.

PROBLEM 92

Lipid-soluble drugs such as thiopental

    a. penetrate fat deposits extensively and rapidly
    b. penetrate fat deposits extensively but slowly
    c. cross the blood brain barrier slowly
    d. do not cross the placenta
    e. are not absorbed from the gastrointestinal tract

Answer   ⒝

Although drugs with the properties of thiopental have a high affinity for fat, they penetrate fat slowly because of the relatively poor blood supply to fat. The lipid blood brain barrier, however, has a very high blood perfusion rate so penetration of the brain is rapid. Lipid solubility facilitates transfer across the placenta and the gastrointestinal membranes.

PROBLEM 93

If a drug has a volume of distribution of approximately 50 l in a 70-kg person, it is probably distributed

    a. only in plasma
    b. only in bone marrow
    c. only in the brain
    d. evenly through body water
    e. evenly through extracellular fluid

Answer   d

Total body water is about five-sevenths of body volume. Plasma, bone marrow, brain, and extracellular fluids are all of lesser volume.

PROBLEM 94

Many drugs undergo biotransformation in the body and these metabolic reactions more often than not

    a. activate the compounds
    b. increase the polarity of the compounds
    c. occur in the kidney
    d. involve either a Phase I or a Phase II reaction
    e. involve a hydrolysis reaction

Answer   b

Generally speaking, biotransformation *removes* activity, occurs in the *liver* more than in the kidney, and involves *both* a Phase I and a Phase II reaction, and hydrolysis is relatively rare. Thus only (b) is a generally correct possibility.

PROBLEM 95

Acetaminophen is metabolized to the structure indicated in Fig. 15. This is

  a. paracetamol
  b. acetaminophenetidin
  c. phenacetin
  d. acetaminophen sulfate
  e. paracetamol glucuronide

Answer   e

It would be possible to present literally hundreds of chemical formulae for identification. This one is given as an example of a type of question useful in testing. Examples used in any context would depend on the drugs mentioned in the relevant courses.

PROBLEM 95

Illustration

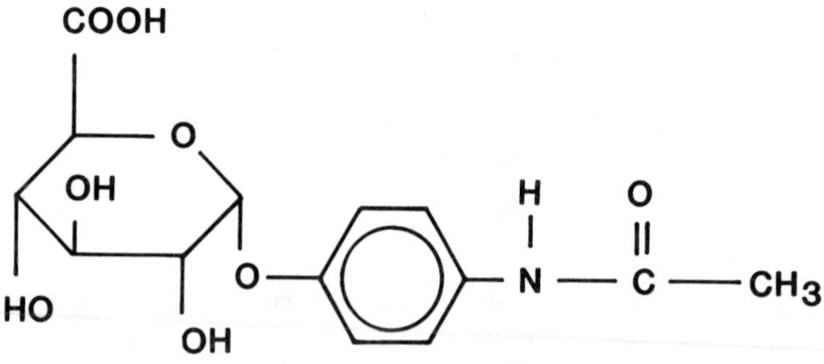

Fig. 15. Chemical structure of one particular acetaminophen metabolite.

PROBLEM 96

If a drug metabolite decays in plasma more slowly than does its precursor,

   a. its decay is limited by its formation and nothing else
   b. its decay is a function of its own elimination rate constant, which will be the same if it is administered in its own right
   c. it must be more protein bound than its precursor
   d. it must have a higher volume of distribution than its precursor
   e. its metabolism must be inhibited by the percursor

Answer   b

The equation for the standard plasma concentration graph seen following oral doses is generally presumed to directly indicate the rate constants of absorption (growth) and elimination (decay). In certain circumstances, notably when liberation from the dosage form controls the rate of transfer of the drug through the body, the decay phase indicates the absorption rate constant and the growth phase indicates the elimination rate constant. A "flip-flop" model is said to apply. Metabolite concentrations also show growth and decay kinetics. This problem highlights the concept of a flip-flop model applied to metabolite kinetics. The metabolite concentration cannot decay more rapidly than that of its precursor, when formed from the precursor (it can decay relatively rapidly if the metabolite itself is administered). If it decays relatively slowly, it is usually because it has a relatively low elimination rate constant. If it decays at the same rate as that of the precursor, it *may* mean that its decay is formation limited (flip-flop case).

PROBLEM 97

If more of a drug is excreted when the urine is acidified metabolically than when the urine is made alkaline metabolically,

   a. the drug is a weak acid and therefore reabsorbed from acidic urine

b. the drug is a weak acid and therefore reabsorbed from alkaline urine
c. the drug is a weak base and therefore reabsorbed from acidic urine
d. the drug is a weak base and therefore reabsorbed from alkaline urine
e. the higher excretion can be caused by ingestion of sodium bicarbonate

Answer   d

Weak acids tend to be excreted more rapidly in alkaline urine because of lesser reabsorption. Weak bases are similarly reabsorbed more from alkaline urine. Thus, only answer (d) can be correct. Bicarbonate causes alkaline urine.

PROBLEM 98

The renal excretion of a drug will be reduced if

a. the drug is a weak acid and the urinary pH is made acid
b. the drug is a weak base and the urinary pH is reduced
c. the drug is an amine, and ammonium chloride is administered
d. the drug is aspirin, and sodium bicarbonate is administered
e. the drug is ethanol, and sodium bicarbonate is administered

Answer   a

Ammonium chloride acidifies urine and sodium bicarbonate has no effect on neutral molecules such as ethanol.

PROBLEM 99

Assuming first-order elimination kinetics, accumulation of a drug in the body during multiple dose regimens

a. occurs over a longer period of time with higher doses
b. results in a decreased rate of elimination
c. continues after attainment of steady state
d. continues for as long as drug is being administered
e. allows for 90% of the steady state to be reached within three half-lives

Answer   d

Answer (a) is not correct because Cp_{ss} depends on dose but is independent of time. Answer (b) is not correct, because as plasma levels increase, with first-order elimination, the rate constant of elimination stays constant but the rate of elimination increases. Answer (c) could not be correct because existence of steady state implies no further accumulation. Answer (e) is not correct because 90% of the steady-state concentration is achieved once $3.32 \times T_{1/2}$ have elapsed. This leaves answer (d) which sounds incorrect. It focuses attention on the fact that a true steady state is not reached until $T = \infty$, but drugs are not given for an infinite time.

PROBLEM 100

In constant intravenous infusion therapy, a priming dose

a. is useful for drugs which have a very long half-life
b. is employed to increase the steady-state concentration
c. will not alter the time required to reach steady state
d. decreases the infusion rate necessary to maintain the desired plasma concentration
e. should be at least ten times the maintenance dose

Answer   a

A priming dose is used to induce a steady-state concentration rapidly, not to change the steady-state concentration. It thus *alters* the time required to reach steady state. It does not decrease the infusion rate needed to maintain the desired concentration, and there is no ten times rule of thumb. Since time to reach steady state is a function of $T_{1/2}$, a priming dose is especially useful with long $T_{1/2}$ drugs.

PROBLEM 101

When a drug normally given every eight hours is changed suddenly to the same daily amount but in a single daily dose.

a. the area under the curve of plasma level of drug against time in the first eight hours of the first 24-hour dosage period is reduced
b. the area under the curve in (a) is increased fourfold
c. the degree of fluctuation between peaks and troughs increases twofold
d. the troughs start to fall below the threshold for effect if the eight-hourly regimen troughs were equal to that threshold
e. the peaks start to rise above the toxicity threshold if the eight-hourly regimen peaks were 0.25 times that threshold

Answer   d

The area under the curve stays the same, the fluctuation increases more than twofold, and the troughs become lower, but the increase in peak concentration is not great enough to lead to an increase above the toxicity threshold.

PROBLEM 102

The dibucaine number

a. assesses acetylator status
b. is obtained with a local anesthetic and acetylcholinesterase and butyrylcholine
c. is obtained with dibucaine, plasma pseudocholinesterase, and succinylcholine
d. is lower in patients who suffer prolonged apnea from succinylcholine treatment
e. is a measure of the ability of the liver to metabolize pseudocholinesterases

Answer   d

The dibucaine number assesses plasma pseudocholinesterase, using butyrylcholine and dibucaine, not acetylcholine. It *is* low in patients who suffer prolonged apnea. The enzyme activity is that in *plasma* not liver.

PROBLEM 103

Sulfamethazine metabolism

    a. assesses acetylator status from data for sulfanilic acid and acetylsulfamethazine

    b. is a guide to isoniazid dosing because slow acetylators are at risk from liver damage

    c. is a guide to sulfonamide dosing because fast acetylators develop peripheral neuritis

    d. indicates that all Eskimos are slow acetylators

    e. assesses the need for caution in prescribing isoniazid because slow acetylators may suffer from pyridoxal deficiencies

Answer [e]

This test uses sulfamethazine not sulfanilic acid. Slow acetylators are protected from liver damage, but are at risk from peripheral neuritis. Eskimos have zero or almost zero incidence of slow acetylation, leaving statement (e) as the only one correct.

PROBLEM 104

The following are generally accepted trends with increasing age:

    a. decreasing drug-conjugating ability of the liver in the first three months of life

    b. an increase in gastric acidity in late middle age

    c. a decrease in creatinine clearance from age 20 onwards at about 1% per year

    d. a gradual decrease in the ampicillin rate constant for elimination of the drug in the first 68 days of life

    e. a gradual increase in digoxin tissue sensitivity as patients go from childhood to adulthood

Answer $\boxed{c}$

Conjugating ability increases during the first three months, gastric acid secretion decreases with age, (c) is correct, ampicillin excretion increases during the first 68 days of life, and children show a relatively high digoxin tissue sensitivity.

PROBLEM 105

Tolbutamide is eliminated more rapidly in hepatitis *principally*

 a. because it has a low volume of distribution and protein binding is lower during hepatitis
 b. because it is a high-extraction drug and plasma albumin is increased during hepatitis
 c. because the blood flow to the liver increases during hepatitis
 d. because it lowers blood sugar
 e. because the kidney takes over its elimination

Answer $\boxed{a}$

Tolbutamide is bound to albumin. It is also a low-extraction-ratio, low-Vd drug and its hepatic clearance is affected by binding. Since binding is reduced in liver disease, and because albumin concentrations fall, it actually shows faster metabolism.

PROBLEM 106

In the various protein binding diagrams available

 a. the double reciprocal plot of Klotz allows calculation of K and n but uses concentration of drug bound in both x and y axes
 b. the plot of Scatchard allows calculation of K and n but is only applicable to data where the identity and concentration of the binding protein is unknown
 c. the plot of Scatchard is immune to the statistical criticisim that extrapolation is bad

d. the plot of Rosenthal allows calculation of K and n when the identity of the binding protein is unknown

e. the plot of Rosenthal allows calculation of K but not n when the concentration of the binding protein is unknown

Answer e

Only (e) is correct, as shown by examination of the theory behind the various plots.

PROBLEM 107

A hyperthyroid patient required phenytoin and propranolol. His phenytoin levels were found to be higher than in euthyroid patients, while his propranolol levels were lower than in euthyroid patients. Which of the following is the most likely explanation?

a. Increased liver blood flow caused relatively fast metabolism of propranolol; phenytoin levels unexplained.

b. Phenytoin increased absorption of propranolol; phenytoin levels unexplained.

c. Phenytoin metabolism increased; propranolol metabolism increased.

d. Phenytoin metabolism increased; propranolol metabolism decreased.

e. Both drugs show a faster rate of absorption in hyperthyroidism.

Answer a

Thyroid conditions alter drug disposition. Hypothyroid conditions lead to slower metabolism, reduced organ perfusion, etc., with the opposite true for hyperthyroid conditions. Thus, (a) is correct because increased liver blood flow is expected and the phenytoin observation fits no principles. There is no well-known effect of phenytoin to increase propranolol absorption; this would in any case increase, not decrease, propranolol concentrations. In (c) and (d) an increase in the rate of metabolism of phenytoin would decrease phenytoin levels. Absorption effects are undocumented, but the same effect on absorption of both drugs would cause a change in plasma levels in the same direction.

PROBLEM 108

Warfarin has a low extraction ratio, a low volume of distribution, and a low free fraction in plasma. According to the Wilkinson–Shand theory of clearance, a decrease in binding to plasma protein will

a. have no effect on hepatic clearance
b. have no effect on total "steady-state" concentrations in plasma (free + bound, Cp_{ss})
c. have no effect on "steady-state" concentration in plasma water (Cp'_{ss})
d. have the same effect on half-life in plasma as would occur with a decrease in binding of propranolol
e. increase the half-life in plasma water, to a relatively small extent because of the low volume of distribution

Answer   [c]

See the explanation of the Wilkinson–Shand equation in Part IV, problem 134, and in Table 1. Propranolol is a drug with a high extraction ratio and, therefore, with properties opposite to those of warfarin.

PROBLEM 109

Phenylbutazone has a low extraction ratio, a low apparent volume of distribution, and a low free fraction in plasma. According to the Wilkinson–Shand theory of clearance, an increase in binding to plasma protein will

a. have no effect on hepatic clearance
b. have no effect on total "steady-state" concentrations in plasma (free + bound)
c. increase "steady-state" concentrations in plasma water

    d. produce a relatively large increase in plasma half-life because of the low volume of distribution

    e. decrease both hepatic clearance and total "steady-state" concentrations

Answer ☐d

According to the Wilkinson–Shand theory, a *decrease* in the binding of a drug with the properties of phenylbutazone will increase hepatic clearance, decrease total steady-state concentrations, have no effect on nonbound (free) steady-state concentrations, and decrease the half-life significantly because of the relatively low apparent volume of distribution. The question seeks the results of an *increase* in binding, so that only (d) can be true.

PROBLEM 110

According to the Wilkinson–Shand theory, in which k_m is the first-order rate constant of metabolism, V_L is the volume of the liver, and P is the partition coefficient of distribution of the drug between liver and blood

    a. $Cl_{intrinsic} = k_m V_L P$

    b. protein-bound drug is metabolized more rapidly

    c. $Cl_{intrinsic} = QE$

    d. f_B = fraction bound

    e. hepatic clearance $= Cl_{intrinsic}/(Q + Cl_{intrinsic})$

Answer ☐a

According to this theory, protein-bound drug is metabolized relatively slowly, whole Cl_H equals QE and $Cl_{intrinsic} = Cl_H$. The original paper uses f_B for fraction *unbound* in *blood*. The equation in (e) defines extraction ratio E.

PROBLEM 111

The Michaelis–Menten equation is most commonly used in pharmacokinetics to describe

a. zero-order first-pass effects
b. nonlinear or dose-dependent elimination of drugs
c. drug accumulation to steady state
d. the total area under the plasma level versus time curve
e. placental transfer of drugs

Answer   ⓑ

Application to dose-dependent elimination is common. Application to absorption is also common, and Michaelis–Menten kinetics are a factor in drug accumulation to steady state in the particular case of phenytoin.

PROBLEM 112

What is the error in the following case study? A gentamicin dose (100 mg) was infused from 9–9:30 A.M. The gentamicin concentration at 45 minutes after starting infusion was 10 μg/ml; the gentamicin concentration eight hours later was 0.1 μg/ml; a decision was made to increase the dose because the trough was low.

a. The analysis was wrong.
b. The original dose was too high.
c. The first sample was collected too early; the dose should not be increased on the basis of trough levels.
d. Gentamicin should not be studied before 12 noon.
e. Gentamicin should be given i.v. push for pharmacokinetic studies.

Answer   ⓒ

Gentamicin is a two- (or perhaps three-) compartment drug. During the first 30 minutes following the *end* of an infusion, the drug concentration declines relatively rapidly as the result of the gradual establishment of equilibrium within the body. It is important, therefore, to delay until at least 30 minutes after the end of the infusion, and possibly until 60 minutes, the collection of the first blood sample, when the clinically applicable half-life is to be estimated from a "peak" and a "trough." The 45-minute point in this problem was 45 minutes after *starting* the 30-minute infusion, or just 15 minutes after its termination.

PROBLEM 113

In a feathering (curve stripping or method of residuals technique) exercise, with a multiexponential decay graph, an underestimate of the rate constant of the terminal decay phase will lead to

    a. a concave line (bowed towards the origin) for the "residual" data
    b. a convex line (bowed away from the original) for the "residual" data
    c. a reduced value for Vd based on the extrapolated construction line
    d. evidence that an extra compartment exists
    e. a reduced calculated terminal phase half-life

Answer   b

An underestimate of the rate constant of the terminal decay phase leads to a line with too shallow a slope and an underestimate of the intercept. The residuals then become relatively large, with an especially great influence when the residuals are small, leading to a convex residual curve. Also, Vd(extrapol.) will be overestimated, there will be no evidence of an extra compartment, and an *increased* terminal phase half-life will result.

PROBLEM 114

If a drug is 99% bound to plasma protein and it is reasonable to assume that the protein concentration is much greater than both the unbound drug concentration and unity, then which of the following is true?

    a. Doubling the number of binding sites (n) per molecule will halve the fraction bound (β).
    b. Halving the protein concentration (Pt) will double the fraction bound (β).
    c. Doubling Pt will double the fraction unbound (α).
    d. Doubling n and halving Pt will leave α unchanged.
    e. Halving the binding equilibrium constant will multiply α by 4.

Answer   [d]

The equation for fraction bound (β) is:

$$\beta = \frac{1}{1 + Df/n\text{Pt} + 1/nK\text{Pt}}$$

where Df is unbound drug concentration, n is the number of binding sites per molecule, Pt is molar protein concentration, and K is the binding constant. Generally speaking, Df is much less than Pt; therefore, Df/nPt tends to zero. Also, nKPt is generally much greater than 1, so

$$\beta = 1 - 1/nK\text{Pt}$$

and since $\alpha = 1 - \beta$,

$$\alpha = 1/nK\text{Pt}$$

From this, doubling n will double β, halving Pt will halve α, doubling Pt will halve α, doubling n and halving Pt will leave α unchanged, and halving K will multiply α by 2.

PROBLEM 115

One of your patients has been prescribed tetracycline, 250 mg every 8 hours. He had taken his first four doses without difficulty, but 4 hours after taking his fifth dose, he vomited. He was not sure whether or not he had lost the capsule, in part or completely. What would you advise?

    a. Take another 250 mg dose immediately, and resume the normal regimen 6 hours later;

    b. Take another 250 mg dose immediately, and resume the normal regimen 8 hours later, with all subsequent doses 2 hours later than originally planned;

    c. Take half a dose immediately, and resume the normal regimen 6 hours later;

    d. Rush the patient to hospital, with a vomit sample, for blood and vomit assays of tetracycline content, with a view to calculating just the right dose to replace any tetracycline lost, then giving that dose by injection;

e. Do nothing until the next 8-hourly dose is needed, then resume the 8-hourly regimen

Answer ☐e

There probably would be no need to do anything. At least some of the tetracycline would have been absorbed and the blood concentration would probably have been comfortably above the minimum inhibitory concentration. While excessive tetracycline causes no problems if given for one dosage interval, there would be no need to compensate what would have been at most a partial loss. In the answers above, (a) and (b) would almost certainly over compensate. Answer (c) would be subtly correct, but probably not worth the effort. Answer (d) would be a gross over-reaction. Consider whether your recommendation would be different if vomiting occurred within 30 minutes of the dose, especially if the capsule dose was detected in the vomited material. Consider also the same circumstances but with different drugs, e.g. theophylline, thyroxine, warfain, digoxin or magnesium hydroxide.

PROBLEM 116

A certain patient had taken two aspirin tablets for a headache. His headache was still present after three hours. He wanted to take more aspirin, but the instructions on the bottle stated that dosing should be no more frequent than every 4 hours. Which of the following courses of action would have led to the highest concentrations of aspirin in the patient's body two hours from the three hour point when the headache was still present? The half-life of aspirin is approximately 30 minutes.

a. Taking one more tablet immediately
b. Waiting one hour, and taking two more tablets
c. Taking one more tablet immediately, then another one one hour later
d. Taking an Advil tablet
e. Taking no more aspirin, but taking ammonium cloride to acidify the urine, so that aspirin excretion occurred more slowly

Answer b

Taking an Advil tablet would add ibuprofen, not more aspirin to the blood. Taking ammonium cloride would slow down aspirin excretion, but would not increase the concentration in plasma above that present at the three hour point in the question. You therefore have to sort out which of (a) (b) and (c) would have the stated effect. Taking two tablets will lead to a greater increase than taking one, so (a) is not correct. In answer (b) during the one hour wait, 75% of the body content will disappear, because of the 30 minute half-life, but this will be 75% of a very small quantity. If one tablet were to be taken immediately, this would also be 75% metabolized during that hour, so waiting one hour and then taking two would achieve the pharmacokinetic objective. Note that clinical and pharmacokinetic objectives may not call for the same action.

PROBLEM 117

A certain patient had been prescribed an antibiotic to be given at 8 A.M., 4 P.M. and 12 midnight. The half-life of the antibiotic was 2 hours, and the prescription was designed to keep the steady-state trough levels at twice the minimum inhibitory concentration (M.I.C.). Toxicity was observable at 35 (or more) times the M.I.C. On the second evening of treatment, at 8 P.M. the patient called, saying that he had missed his 4 P.M. dose. Which of the following possible courses of action would be best?

    a. Wait until midnight and resume dosing
    b. Take the 4 P.M. dose immediately and resume the normal schedule at midnight
    c. Take the 4 P.M. dose immediately and thereafter take doses at 4 A.M., 12 noon, and 8 P.M.
    d. Break a tablet in half, take one half immediately, and resume the normal schedule at midnight
    e. Take no more tablets until 8 A.M., then obtain a whole new supply, and start all over again

Answer d

With an 8 hour dosing interval and a half-life of 2 hours, fluctuation at steady state involves 16-fold increases from trough to peak, and

93.75% falls from peak to trough. Since troughs are twice the M.I.C., toxicity occurs at 17.5 times the troughs $(35 \div 2)$, just above the peaks. At 8 P.M. the concentration was at 0.5 times the M.I.C. A four hour wait (to midnight) could be therapeutically disastrous. However, a full dose at 8 P.M. would give a midnight trough of 3.8 times the desired trough, leading to a peak above the toxic level. Answer (c) would be inconvenient, although therapeutically satisfactory. Waiting until 8 A.M. would be more unsatisfactory than waiting until midnight. Taking half a tablet would raise the concentration above the M.I.C. It would then fall by 75% by midnight, when resumption of 8-hourly dosing would keep the peaks low enough and the troughs high enough.

PROBLEM 118

Diclofenac sodium is a non-steroidal antiinflammatory agent. When given every 12 hours, it is "completely" cleared from blood with a half-life of less than 3 hours. However, it is found in joint fluid longer. Pharmacokinetically speaking, this means:

   a. that diclofenac sodium has a relatively long half-life in joint fluid
   b. that diclofenac sodium is a two-compartment drug, with joint fluid behaving as a peripheral compartment
   c. that diclofenac sodium is preferentially localized in joint fluid, so that the relatively high concentrations are more easily detected
   d. that joint fluid is more alkaline than blood
   e. that diclofenac sodium is better than other non-steroidal antiinflammatory drugs

Answer   ⒞

Answer (a) is not correct, as the half-life values in joint fluid and in-plasma could be the same, with the concentrations in plasma having dropped below detection limits. Answer (b) is not correct, as tissue concentrations exceeding plasma concentrations do not, as such, indicate two compartment cases. Answer (d) is not indicated, although relatively alkaline tissue fluid would indeed attract diclofenac. Answer (e) is a non-sequiter, leaving answer (c) as the only one correct.

PROBLEM 119

A certain patient had a history of delayed gastric emptying and less than normal peristalsis. She needed a systematic antibiotic to treat a bronchial infection. The antibiotic was usually given orally as a loading dose followed by maintenance doses. Compared with the normal population, which of the following would you recommend?

    a. The usual dosage
    b. A larger loading dose than usual with smaller maintenance doses
    c. A smaller loading dose than usual, with larger maintenance doses
    d. An intramuscular loading dose followed by the usual maintenance doses
    e. The usual dosage regimen plus a gastrointestinal stimulant

Answer   d

This patient would react relatively slowly to the initial doses if given orally. Thus the usual dosage (a) would be relatively inefficient. A larger loading dose might be a good idea, but not with smaller maintenance doses (b). A smaller loading dose would be nonsensical, even with larger maintenance doses (c). Use of a gastrointestinal stimulant, whatever that is, would be a poor approach, as it would add the unpredictability of a drug interaction. Answer (d) is a good one.

PART IV:
Multiple Answer
Factual Questions

In this part of the book, one or more answers in each question are correct. Follow the usual code:

Answer a if 1, 2, and 3 are correct.
Answer b if 1 and 3 are correct.
Answer c if 2 and 4 are correct.
Answer d if only 4 is correct.
Answer e if all are correct.

PROBLEM 120

In the equation $\ln Cp_t = \ln Cp_0 - k_{el}t$

1. $\ln Cp_0 = 2.303 \log Cp_0$

2. $k_{el} = \dfrac{0.693}{T_{1/2}}$

3. $Cp_0 = \dfrac{\text{Dose}}{\text{Vd}}$

4. ln indicates logarithm to base 10

Answer [a]

The practice of clinical pharmacokinetics requires the ability to read an equation, to immediately perceive its message, and, when appropriate, to visualize the shape of the relationship resulting when two of the symbols are related as variables x and y on graph paper. This and the next three problems are concerned with this skill. All of the equations are taken from the introductory section of this book. In this particular problem, statements, 1, 2, and 3 are correct, so that the correct answer to the problem is (a).

PROBLEM 121

In the equation $Cp_t = Cp_0 \exp(-k_{el}t)$

1. C indicates concentration
2. exp and the symbols following it indicate the same as e raised to the power $(-k_{el}t)$
3. p indicates that the measurement was made in plasma
4. k_{el} is a first-order rate constant

Answer [e]

All four are correct.

PROBLEM 122

In the equation $\dfrac{dQd}{dt} = k_0 - k_{el}Qd$

1. the expression describes the rate of change of the amount of drug in a biological system into which the drug is introduced by zero-order infusion
2. k_0 is the rate constant of infusion
3. Cp could be substituted for Qd, if Vd was constant, without changing the shape of the graph described
4. the equation describes a graph showing concentration decreasing at a gradually increasing rate until a plateau is reached

Answer a

Answers 1, 2, and 3 are correct. Answer 4 is incorrect because of the reference to concentration decreasing. The equation is for a rate of change of a quantity in the body. Its integrated form, with correction for volume of distribution, would describe a concentration *increasing* at a gradually decreasing rate.

PROBLEM 123

In the equation $Cp_t = \dfrac{FD}{Vd} \cdot \dfrac{k_a}{k_a - k_{el}} (e^{-k_{el}t} - e^{-k_a t})$

1. F represents the fraction excreted unchanged
2. D stands for drug
3. Vd is the reciprocal of clearance
4. $\dfrac{FD}{Vd} \cdot \dfrac{k_a}{k_a - k_{el}} = Cp_0$

Answer d

Letters a, F, D, and Vd stand for absorption, fraction absorbed, dose, and apparent volume of distribution, respectively.

PROBLEM 124

The conventional equation for renal clearance

1. is $Cl = \dfrac{Cu}{Cp} \times V$
2. evaluates the volume of plasma from which the drug is totally removed by the kidneys in unit time
3. defines a clearance of over 130 ml/min as indicating net transfer of the drug in question from renal tubular blood into the renal tubule
4. allows no correction for protein binding

Answer [e]

All four are correct.

PROBLEM 125

The equation for Michaelis–Menten kinetics

1. relates the measured rate of reaction, the maximum possible rate of the reaction, the substrate concentration, and a constant
2. is especially suitable to phenytoin (dilantin) kinetics
3. is likely to be applicable to plasma concentration data deviating from straight-line decay when graphed on both linear and log-linear coordinates
4. reduces to a zero-order expression at low substrate concentrations

Answer [a]

Answers 1, 2, and 3 are correct. The Michaelis–Menten equation reduces to a first-order expression at low substrate concentrations and to a zero-order expression at high substrate concentrations.

PROBLEM 126

If a drug concentration decays in two phases following an intravenous bolus injection,

1. the half-time of decay of the second phase is commonly called the β-phase half-life
2. the effect will decrease as the concentration falls if the drug receptors are in the central compartment
3. total body clearance $= Vd \cdot \beta$
4. the effect will decrease as the concentration falls during the faster phase of decay if the drug receptors are in the peripheral compartment

Answer [a]

Statements 1, 2, and 3 are correct, but statement 4 is incorrect; the effect will increase during the α-phase, which is dominated by drug distribution into the peripheral compartment.

PROBLEM 127

If a dose is doubled and absorption, distribution, and elimination processes follow first-order kinetics and show no dose-dependent or time-dependent changes,

1. t_{max} stays the same
2. the intensity of effect doubles if effect and log dose are linearly related
3. Cp at t_{max} doubles
4. the duration of effect doubles if effect and log dose are linearly related

Answer [b]

Every pharmacokineticist should be able to express in words what happens to the single-dose, first-order absorption/elimination growth and decay curve when k_a, k_{el}, F, D, etc., are changed singly or together. The relevant relationships for intensity and duration of effect should also be understood.

PROBLEM 128

First-order kinetics

1. means the rate of reaction is proportional to concentration
2. is more common than zero-order kinetics
3. applies to exponential processes
4. results in steady-state concentrations after multiple dosing

Answer [e]

These are simple definition statements concerned with the basic features of first-order kinetics. All four are correct.

PROBLEM 129

Single-compartment open model means that

1. the drug is restricted to extracellular fluid
2. the drug does not penetrate tissues
3. the drug is highly ionized
4. one exponential term describes a decreasing plasma concentration of the drug when kinetics are first order

Answer [d]

The number of compartments reflects our ability to subdivide the body on the basis of delivery rates of drugs to tissues, not on the basis of actual body spaces. Ionization has nothing to do with the matter.

PROBLEM 130

Drug absorption of weak acids such as aspirin

1. occurs by diffusion of the nonionized form
2. is accelerated by alkalinization of the stomach

3. would occur more slowly if the drugs were not bound to plasma protein
4. stops if the aspirin is formulated with sodium bicarbonate and tartaric acid

Answer   b̄

Extensive studies with various weak electrolyte drugs have resulted in a pH–partition hypothesis of drug absorption. This hypothesis is described in all of the relevant textbooks. The facts are: (a) nonionized forms of weak electrolyted diffuse relatively easily through membranes (b) weak acids are more ionized at relatively high pH values, and (c) weak bases are more ionized at relatively low pH values. The fact that statements 1 and 3 are correct then follows from basic principles, with the added influence of protein binding in plasma increasing the concentration gradient, and therefore the rate of absorption, between the gastrointestinal lumen and plasma water.

PROBLEM 131

Binding of drugs to plasma protein

1. is usually expressed as the fraction or percentage bound
2. is a major influence on the volume of distribution
3. is never inversely proportional to protein concentration
4. involves albumin exclusively

Answer   ā

Binding of drugs to plasma protein can be evaluated by means of the equilibrium constant (K), the number of binding sites per molecule (n), and the fraction or percentage bound (β). The commonest clinical expression is of β. Binding is a major influence on the volume of distribution and is proportional to protein concentration in certain circumstances but is never inversely proportional to protein concentration. Protein binding involves several proteins other than albumin.

PROBLEM 132

Salicylic acid is a metabolite of acetylsalicylic acid; salicylic acid has the longer half-life (it actually commonly shows Michaelis–Menten kinetics). After an intravenous dose of acetylsalicylic acid, the following half-life values were obtained: $T_{1/2}$ for decline of acetylsalicylic acid concentration in plasma, 0.5 h; $T_{1/2}$ for increase of salicylic acid concentrations in plasma, 0.5 h; $T_{1/2}$ for decrease in salicylic acid concentrations in plasma, 5 h. What can you logically conclude?

1. Salicylic acid is converted to aspirin in the body.
2. A flip-flop model is not applicable to the salicylic acid concentrations.
3. Salicylic acid inhibits acetylsalicylic acid metabolism.
4. Acetylsalicylic acid is converted to salicylic acid and nothing else.

Answer   ©

Although metabolism facilitates excretion, drug metabolites commonly persist in the body for longer than do their parent drugs. Indeed, the absolute maximum rate of metabolite elimination is the same as that of its precursor (except when the metabolite is itself administered, as opposed to being formed from its parent drug). In certain circumstances, the kinetics of decay of the metabolite formation, when a flip-flop model is said to apply. In this problem, the metabolite decays more slowly than does the precursor, and the rate constant of increase of the metabolite concentration is the same as that of decrease of the precursor. A conventional (not a flip-flop) model therefore applies. Statements 2 and 4 are logically true on the basis of the evidence presented.

PROBLEM 133

When a drug metabolite B is formed from a drug A,

1. in spite of greater polarity of B compared with A, it is possible for B to persist in the body longer than A

2. there are no circumstances in which plasma levels of B can decline faster than those of A
3. the rate constant of formation of the metabolite is the same as the rate constant of disappearance of A when no other formation or elimination processes are involved
4. when the rate constant of formation of B is less than the rate constant of elimination of B [and the conditions in (3) apply] the disappearances of A and B from plasma occur at the same rate

Answer [e]

This problem should be approached by means of visualization, or even sketching, of different possible relationships between kinetics of decay of parent drug and kinetics of growth and decay of metabolite. All four statements are correct.

PROBLEM 134

According to the Wilkinson–Shand equation, an increase in binding to plasma protein

1. has no effect on the hepatic clearance of a drug with a high intrinsic clearance
2. increases total steady-state concentrations of low-extraction-ratio drugs
3. has no effect on steady-state concentrations of unbound drug, for low-extraction-ratio drugs
4. causes a decrease in the half-life of high-extraction-ratio drugs

Answer [d]

The Wilkinson–Shand equation expresses the relation between hepatic clearance, hepatic blood flow, protein binding, and a characteristic of the drug in question, its intrinsic clearance in the liver. On the basis of this equation, it is possible to make a statement concerning the likely effect of protein binding changes on hepatic clearance and steady-state concentrations, as well as on other measurements, depending on the characteristics of the drug.

Table 1. Anticipated effect of an increase in binding to plasma protein on certain pharmacokinetic variables assuming the "well-stirred" liver model

Extraction ratio (E)	Hepatic clearance (Cl_H)	Steady-state concentration in plasma (Cp_{ss})	Steady-state concentration in plasma water (Cp'_{ss})	Half-life in plasma ($T_{1/2}$)
High	None	None	Decrease	If Vd high, relatively large decrease
				If Vd low, relatively small decrease
Low	Decrease	Increase	None	If Vd high, relatively small increase
				If Vd low, relatively large increase

The predictions are summarized in Table 1, use of which in relation to this question reveals only statement 4 to be correct.

PROBLEM 135

According to the Wilkinson–Shand approach to protein binding and clearance, an increase in the bound fraction of a drug distributed through a one-compartment system leads to

1. an increase in the hepatic clearance of a low-extraction-ratio drug
2. an increase in the mean Cp_{ss} of total drug in plasma with no effect on the mean Cp_{ss} of unbound drug in plasma for a drug with the properties of warfarin
3. a decrease in the half-life of drug concentration in plasma for a drug with the properties of warfarin
4. a decrease in the hepatic clearance of drug with a low E value

Answer   c

See the explanations to the previous two questions. In this problem, statements 2 and 4 are correct. The low-extraction-ratio drug will show a decrease in hepatic clearance with an increase in fraction bound. Warfarin is a low-extraction-ratio drug (low E value).

PROBLEM 136

According to the Wilkinson–Shand equation,

1. hepatic clearance is a function of hepatic blood flow and intrinsic clearance
2. extraction ratio = intrinsic clearance/(hepatic blood flow + intrinsic clearance)
3. when the extraction ratio is relatively high, hepatic clearance = hepatic blood flow
4. when the extraction ratio is relatively low, hepatic clearance = intrinsic clearance

Answer   b

See the last three questions for notes on the Wilkinson–Shand equation. In this question, statements 1 and 3 are correct.

PROBLEM 137

According to the theory which treats renal excretion as comprising two sequential "single pool" equilibria (i.e., one at the glomerulus and a second in the renal tubule),

1. an increase in renal blood flow will decrease renal clearance in all circumstances
2. protein binding will retain an influence regardless of the relationship between renal blood flow and intrinsic renal tubular clearance
3. renal clearance increases with increased urine flow rate
4. creatinine clearance appears in the formula for definition of renal clearance

Answer   c

The relevant definition of renal clearance is:

$$Cl_R = \left[Cl_{cr} + \frac{Q_K Cl'_T}{Q_K + \alpha\, Cl'_T} \right]$$

where Cl_{cr} is creatinine clearance, Q_K is renal blood flow, Cl'_T is an intrinsic renal tubular clearance for unbound drug, and α is the free fraction in plasma. Examination of statements 1 and 4 in relation to this equation shows that only statements 2 and 4 are correct. Statement 3 happens to be true as a statement of fact, but it is not permitted to occur within the restrictions of this model.

PROBLEM 138

Renal excretion of weak bases such as meperidine

1. is slowed by lowering the pH of urine
2. is accelerated by acidification of urine
3. is accelerated by sodium bicarbonate
4. is generally not affected by inhibitors of active transport

Answer   boxed{c}

Statements 2 and 4 are correct. Statement 1 would be correct if "lowering" was raising, and statement 4 does not apply to drugs which diffuse.

PROBLEM 139

If a drug with a half-life of 24 h is administered as a single daily dose, at steady state the rise and fall in concentrations resulting from the pulsed nature of multiple dosing will result in approximately

1. a doubling after each dose and a 100% decrease from peak to trough
2. a 50% increase after each dose and a 50% decrease from peak to trough
3. more fluctuation than if the dosing interval was 48 h

4. a 100% increase after each dose and a 50% decrease from peak to trough

Answer ⒟

When the dosing interval τ = the half-life ($T_{1/2}$), then the fall from peak to trough is a 50% decrease. Since the problem refers to steady state, the increase must restore the original peak, a doubling or 100% increase. To increase fluctuation, we increase the ratio $\tau/T_{1/2}$. Thus only answer 4 can be correct.

PROBLEM 140

During multiple oral drug dosing,

1. with no loading dose, the plasma concentration will rise towards a "steady state," reaching 90% of this state within $5 \times T_{1/2}$, provided first-order kinetics apply to elimination
2. at "steady state" the rise in plasma concentration resulting from each dose will lead to a doubling of the concentration when the dosage interval is equal to $T_{1/2}$
3. when an appropriate loading dose is given first, the "steady-state" concentration will be established immediately
4. when zero-order elimination kinetics apply, no "steady state" will be achieved

Answer ⒠

This problem should be approached by means of visualization or sketching of the relationships considered. Statement 1 concerns the standard oral dose version of the infusion to steady-state pattern. Statement 2 is concerned with the relation between half-life and dosing interval. Statement 3 is concerned with loading doses. Statement 4 poses the previously unconsidered problem of zero-order elimination kinetics. All four are correct.

PROBLEM 141

During multiple i.v. dosing into a one-compartment system,

1. with no loading dose, the plasma concentration will show an overall rise towards a "steady-state," reaching 99% of this state within $7 \times T_{1/2}$
2. at "steady-state," and after switching to equivalent oral dosing, the rise in plasma concentration resulting from each dose will lead to a doubling of the concentration when the dosage interval is equal to $T_{1/2}$
3. if the following holds true

$$\text{Maintenance Dose} = \text{Loading Dose} \times [1 - \exp(-k_{el})]$$

   the loading dose will institute the steady-state concentration expected from the maintenance dose given alone
4. after switching to oral dosing, the area under the curve within one dosage interval is equal to $\text{Dose}/k_{el}\text{Vd}$

Answer $\boxed{e}$

This problem is similar to the previous one except that it focuses attention on mathematics relevant to loading doses, and also in the area under the curve. All four statements are correct.

PROBLEM 142

If a drug has a first-order rate constant of decay of concentration in the body of $0.0693\,\text{h}^{-1}$, over 90% of the dose will be lost from the body within the following times from the dose:

1. 60 h
2. 50 h
3. 40 h
4. 30 h

Answer $\boxed{a}$

If the rate constant is $0.0693\,\text{h}^{-1}$, the half-life is 10 h. Ninety percent of the dose is lost in $3.32 \times T_{1/2} = 33.2\,\text{h}$, so statements 1, 2, and 3 are all correct. Everything hangs on the word *within*.

PROBLEM 143

Naproxen has a half-life of approximately 13 hours. A patient was planning a move to Saudi Arabia from the U.S.A., with a 7-hour time change. He was trying to work out how to adjust the timing of his naproxen doses so that his peaks and troughs would stay the same during and after his move, so that his mean rate of dosing (mg/h) would stay the same during the changeover and doses would not be needed in the middle of the night in Saudi Arabia. The flying time was 12 hours. Four of his friends offered suggestions. Which of the four (one or more) were logical?

1. Shorten each dosage interval by one hour for $3\frac{1}{2}$ days after arrival in Saudi Arabia and then resume the 12-hour interval.
2. Take an extra full dose on landing in Saudi Arabia.
3. Miss a dose, wait seven hours, and then start a new sequence of 12-hourly dosing.
4. Take a half-tablet six hours after the last dose in the U.S.A., then start a new sequence of 12-hourly dosing.

Answer   ⓓ

Statement 1 is incorrect because it would involve doses during the night in Saudi Arabia, as well as a slight elevation in total dose. Statement 2 is incorrect because it would increase the daily exposure, and statement 3 is incorrect for the same reason. Thus only statement 4 complies with the requirement to maintain an unchanged average rate of dosing expressed as mg/h.

PROBLEM 144

Which of the following statements are true?

1. A graph of intensity of response against dose *in vitro* is hyperbolic.
2. A graph of intensity of response against log dose *in vitro* is sigmoid.
3. Responses are described as "quantal" when only the incidence of response can be measured.

4. "Rate" and "occupancy" theories of drug–receptor interaction lead to very different dose–response relationships.

Answer   [a]

An understanding of dose–response relationships traditionally associated with receptor pharmacology is essential for an understanding of the intensity and duration of drug action *in vivo*, and hence in understanding the relation between pharmacokinetics and pharmacodynamics. In this case, statements 1, 2, and 3 are correct, but statement 4 is the opposite of fact. "Incidence of response" refers to the fact that in some pharmacological systems, only whether or not a response occurs can be measured. The obvious example of this is death in LD_{50} studies. It is then standard practice to calculate the incidence or percentage of occurrence of the standard response (e.g., 70% dead) in a group of responding units, such as a population of small animals.

PROBLEM 145

Assuming that the central portion of the log dose/effect curve is a straight line,

1. intensity of effect *in vivo* declines at a constant rate
2. duration of effect is directly proportional to plasma level
3. duration of effect is directly proportional to log i.v. dose
4. duration of effect is directly proportional to concentration of nonbound drug

Answer   [b]

The answer to this comes direct from the introductory section of this book. Statements 1 and 3 are correct.

PROBLEM 146

Restricting attention to the central portion of a graph of response against log dose and assuming linearity of this portion of the graph with a slope of b and assuming distribution of the drug in question through a single compartment, it can be shown that after an i.v. dose the intensity (I) of effect

1. declines at a constant rate with the slope of a graph of I against time of $k_{el}b/2.303$, if the drug concentration declines exponentially with a rate constant of decline equal to k_{el}
2. declines exponentially
3. declines with zero-order kinetics
4. is affected by the rate constant of transfer of drug between tissues and plasma

Answer ⬛b⬛

Statements 1 and 3 are correct. Statement 2 is incompatible with statements 1 and 3 and statement 4 is just not true.

PROBLEM 147

Making the same assumption as in the previous question, but varying the dose,

1. the duration of effect doubles with each doubling of the dose
2. a plot of duration of effect against dose has an intercept of (log Cp_t)Vd
3. the conclusions apply to d-tubocurarine but not succinylcholine
4. a plot of duration of effect against log i.v. dose is linear with a slope of $2.303/k_{el}$

Answer ⬛d⬛

Statement 1 is known to be incorrect from general knowledge. The conclusions only apply to drugs showing one-compartment distribution. This applies with succinylcholine but not d-tubocurarine.

PROBLEM 150

In the interaction between oral anticoagulants and anti-inflam-
matory drugs

1. phenylbutazone displaces warfarin from binding sites on
   albumin
2. the plasma concentration of warfarin is reduced
3. tissue concentrations of warfarin increase
4. aspirin-induced gastrointestinal bleeding is aggravated

Answer   [a]

Statement 1 is true, as are statements 2 and 3. The tissue levels
increase because warfarin transfers from albumin binding sites to
tissue stores. There is no evidence that statement 4 is true.

PROBLEM 151

In the interaction between oral anticoagulants and phenobarbital

1. phenobarbital withdrawal causes clotting
2. tissue concentrations of warfarin increase while plasma
   concentrations decline
3. the metabolism of phenobarbital is stimulated
4. phenobarbital treatment causes an increase in the concentration of P-450 in the liver

Answer   [d]

Phenobarbital withdrawal leads to slower metabolism of warfarin,
higher plasma warfarin levels, and greater effect (bleeding).
Phenobarbital stimulates the metabolism of warfarin, reducing both
tissue and plasma levels. There is no effect on phenobarbital
metabolism. This leaves statement 4 as the only correct one.

PROBLEM 148

When second and later doses are administered at the moment(s) the effects of their predecessors cease the durations of the effect of the second and later doses are

1. equal to each other but different from that of the first dose
2. different from each other with one of them equal to that of the first dose
3. equal to each other and greater than that of the first dose
4. both double that of the first dose

Answer ⓑ

Answers 1 and 3 are correct. This problem should be solved using a visualization or sketch. If the second dose is administered when the plasma drug concentration has fallen to the theshold level for useful effect, then the second dose builds on a body residue, so that the concentration remains above the threshold for a longer time. If the third dose is given when the second dose "wears-off", its duration will be the same as that of the second dose. Note that all doses are of equal size.

PROBLEM 149

In the interaction between probenecid and penicillin

1. penicillin excretion is slowed
2. probenecid excretion is accelerated
3. uric acid levels in blood are lowered
4. protein binding of penicillin is reduced

Answer ⓑ

Statements 1 and 3 are correct, since probenecid inhibits tabular secretion of penicillin and tubular reabsorption of uric acid.

PROBLEM 152

In the interaction between vasoconstrictor agents and local anesthetics

1. epinephrine aids delivery of lidocaine to its site of action
2. polypeptide vasoconstrictors cause an increase in heart rate
3. procaine amide action is prolonged
4. the vasoconstrictor delays diffusion of the local anesthetic away from the site of injection

Answer ⒟

Epinephrine aids retention of the local anesthetic at its site of action, not delivery to the site. Polypeptide vasoconstrictors lack effects on heart rate. Procaine amide is not administered as a local anesthetic. This leaves statement 4 as the only correct one.

PROBLEM 153

Concurrent consumption of mineral oil and warfarin leads to unusual plasma levels of warfarin. If mineral oil reduces the area under the plasma level vs. time curve of warfarin without affecting the rate constant of growth of plasma levels, and with no increase in the rate constant of decay of plasma levels, the mechanism of interaction could be

1. a slowing of absorption
2. an increase in the rate of elimination
3. a decrease in the rate of elimination
4. a decrease in the extent of absorption

Answer ⒟

The question indicates that answer 1 cannot be correct. Answer 3 cannot be correct because of the word *decrease*. All other things being equal, the area under the curve generally indicates the extent of absorption (answer 4 correct). Strictly speaking, answer 2 could be correct in relation to first-pass metabolism, but a change in the rate constant of decay of plasma levels would also be expected.

PROBLEM 154

If the plasma half-life of antipyrine is decreased as the result of the influence of an interacting drug, the interacting drug most likely

1. increased the concentration of microsomal P-450 in the liver
2. caused faster renal tubular reabsorption of unmetabolized antipyrine
3. is an enzyme inducer
4. caused decreased clearance (as measured from plasma level decay) of antipyrine

Answer   b

If the plasma half-life is decreased, the drug is being eliminated more rapidly. Answers 1 and 3 are clearly possible explanations. Answer 2 cannot be correct because faster *reabsorption* would cause slower elimination. Answer 4 describes the situation of a longer $T_{1/2}$.

PROBLEM 155

In the interaction between phenobarbital and phenytoin (dilantin)

1. phenobarbital concentrations in blood are reduced
2. phenytoin concentrations in blood are reduced
3. the role of each drug in protecting against convulsions is reduced
4. animal experiments suggests liver mass increases

Answer   e

Phenobarbital and phenytoin interfere with each other, but coexist harmoniously. Both stimulate drug-metabolizing enzymes so both are metabolized relatively rapidly, giving reduced plasma concentrations when administered together, although at the same time they compete with each other for the enzymes. As a result, they each reduce the anticonvulsant activity of the other, although the sum of the two together is better in some cases than either one on its own. Enzyme induction results in an increase in liver weight. Thus all four statements are correct.

PROBLEM 156

When amitriptyline is given as a single dose with and without pretreatment with cimetidine, the cimetidine causes increased amitriptyline concentrations and decreased concentrations of nortriptyline formed from the amitriptyline. The $T_{1/2}$ of plasma level decay and the times of maximum concentration are unchanged. What can you conclude?

    1. The first-pass metabolism of amitriptyline to nortriptyline is slowed by cimetidine.
    2. The k_a of amitriptyline is unaffected.
    3. Higher steady-state concentrations of amitriptyline are likely in patients treated with cimetidine.
    4. Protein binding of amitriptyline has changed.

Answer   [a]

There is no evidence in the information given for a protein binding change. The other three statements are plausible conclusions on the basis of the information given.

PROBLEM 157

Which of the following statements concerning interactions between diazepam and other drugs are true?

    1. Cimetidine raises the half-life of diazepam.
    2. Diazepam elevates digoxin levels.

3. Diazepam diminishes the antiparkinsonian effect of levodopa.
4. The combination of lithium carbonate and diazepam can lead to hypothermia.

Answer e

There is an extensive literature concerned with the interactions of diazepam and other drugs. The four statements given are correct.

PROBLEM 158

Patients who are slow acetylators of isoniazid

1. are expecially likely to suffer from peripheral neuritis
2. accumulate N-acetylisoniazid in their blood
3. are also likely to be slow acetylators of procaine amide
4. have excessive quantities of N-acetyltransferase

Answer a

In these patients isoniazid accumulates in plasma to unusually high concentrations, causing depletion of pyridoxal stores and peripheral neuritis. The same enzyme affects procaine amide. In fact, N-acetylisoniazid still accumulates, so that the only incorrect statement is statement 4.

PROBLEM 159

The dibucaine number

1. assesses plasma pseudocholinesterases
2. is obtained by inhibition of benzoylcholine metabolism by dibucaine
3. is useful in predicting responses to succinylcholine
4. is lower in patients with atypical enzymes

Answer e

The dibucaine number was presented as a numerical problem in Part II. See problem 77 for details. In this question, all four statements are correct.

PROBLEM 160

The sulfamethazine acetylation test

1. assesses *N*-acetyltransferase activity
2. involves a test dose of sulfamethazine and measurement of isoniazid in blood
3. indicates that approximately half of all Caucasians are slow acetylators
4. helps prevent liver damage

Answer   ⓑ

The sulfamethazine acetylation test was presented as a numerical problem in Part II. See problem 77 for details. In this question, statements 1 and 3 are correct. Statement 2 is incorrect because isoniazid is not measured, although the test is used in prediction of isoniazid dosing requirements.

PROBLEM 161

Patients likely to experience unusually prolonged apnea when treated with succinylcholine (suxemethonium)

1. have low concentrations of acetylcholinesterase in their livers
2. have atypical pseudocholinesterases in their blood
3. have weak chest muscles
4. can usually be detected in advance by means of a dibucaine number test

Answer   ⓒ

The atypical pseudocholinesterase is synthesized in the liver but is effective in blood; it metabolizes succinylcholine relatively slowly, and its activity is assessed using the dibucaine number.

PROBLEM 162

Which of the following statements are true?

1. The ratio daily dose/steady-state concentration in plasma is relatively high at low daily doses for drugs exhibiting saturable metabolism kinetics.
2. Renal clearance can be urine flow dependent above and beyond the correction for dilution inherent in the formula $Cl = UV/P$.
3. Renal excretion of phenobarbital is relatively sensitive to pH changes, compared with that of pentobarbital and secobarbital, because of the relatively low lipid solubility of phenobarbital.
4. Indocyanine green clearance is used to evaluate hepatic blood flow; antipyrine is used to evaluate microsomal drug metabolizing enzyme activity in the liver.

Answer ⓔ

This problem tests a group of miscellaneous drug disposition facts. All four statements are true, but some thought is needed to determine why they are true. With saturable metabolism, a greater proportion of a small dose is metabolized in unit time, leading to a relatively large proportionate dose demand for given concentrations. Renal clearance *is* greater at high urine flow rates in that the kidney becomes more efficient. Statement 3 is true, and more true than any analogous statements about pK_a values. Indocyanine green and antipyrine are two commonly used research drugs.

PROBLEM 163

Which of the following general mechanisms can be invoked to explain *decreased* drug absorption on administration with a meal?

1. Increase in drug solution due to the pH change caused by the ingested meal, with a resultant increase in the degradation of the susceptible drug, thereby decreasing bioavailability

2. Competition for absorption between the drug and a chemical constituent of the ingested food with the food constituent being preferentially absorbed
3. Prolonged retention of drug in the acidic environment of the stomach due to ingestion of a fatty meal, resulting in increased chemical degradation of the susceptible drug on prolonged exposure to the acid pH
4. Decreased drug solution due to increased viscosity of the stomach contents and consequent inability of dissolved drug to diffuse to the absorption site, thereby decreasing bioavailability

Answer   e

All four are correct.

PROBLEM 164

Which of the following general mechanisms can be invoked to explain *increased* drug absorption on administration with a meal?

1. Decreased first-pass metabolism due to an increase in the splanchic blood flow resulting in increased systemic bioavailability
2. Slower gastric emptying leading to slower delivery of drug to its specific absorption site in the intestine, resulting in lack of saturation of the drug absorption carrier molecule
3. Increase in the peristaltic movements of the gastrointestinal tract, with a resultant increase in the agitation of the drug formulation and the food, thereby aiding drug dissolution for insoluble drugs
4. Increase in the bile flow, with its surfactant-like solubilizing properties enhancing drug dissolution

Answer   e

All four are correct.

PROBLEM 165

Renal impairment

1. can be assessed by blood creatinine measurements
2. causes accumulation of polar metabolites of lipid-soluble drugs
3. can be caused by certain drugs
4. is a factor to be considered in deciding on digoxin dosing

Answer [e]

All four are correct.

PROBLEM 166

What is the error in the following digoxin case study? A 51-year-old female patient was subject to cardiac arrhythmias which were controlled by digoxin. A measurement was made of her digoxin level one morning, approximately three hours following a dose. The level was within the therapeutic range. The clinical pharmacist made the following recommendations and conclusions:

1. check the digoxin level one month later
2. that there were no digoxin-induced unwanted drug effects evident
3. that the patient was taking her tablets
4. that the system was working well

Answer [c]

Statements 1 and 3 are reasonable conclusions, although the data chosen for the next check is entirely arbitrary. Statement 2 implies that the pharmacist was recommending treatment based on levels, not on patient characteristics. A level within the therapeutic range does not imply that no unwanted effects are occurring. Answer 4 is not correct because the sampling time was not optimal. Digoxin sampling times should be delayed until 6–12 h post-dosage because digoxin is a two-compartment drug, and the receptors are in the compartment with the lesser rate of penetration of the drug. Monitoring should be based on levels obtained after intercompartmental equilibration is achieved.

PROBLEM 167

What is the error in the following lithium case study. A 44-year-old male patient has been treated with lithium over a period of five years, during which his serum creatinine had slowly risen. His serum lithium was measured in two samples collected two hours post-dosage on the same day. One sample contained 0.1 mEq/l; the level in the other sample was too high to evaluate. It emerged that the samples had been collected in different tubes, in that 0.1 mEq/l had been recorded in a tube with no anticoagulant, while the other tube had contained heparin as an anticoagulant. The clinical pharmacist was in a dilemma, so he arranged:

1. collection of another sample, ensuring that serum, not plasma, was collected
2. a change in the lithium sampling time to 8–12 h post-dosage in his hospital
3. a check on the analytical methods with "spiked" samples
4. an increase in the lithium dosing because of the low but plausible reading

Answer   d

Answers 1, 2, and 3 describe "good deeds." The high reading was probably obtained because of the use of the lithium salt of heparin. This obviously leads to erroneously high readings. The change to the conventional time of 8–12 h post-dosage would have eased comparison with literature values. A check on the analytical methods is always a good idea. The mistake was to immediately react to the low reading of 0.1. The patient had evidence of kidney damage (serum creatinine) caused by lithium. This could worsen with higher lithium concentrations, so a hasty decision to raise the dose was inappropriate.

PROBLEM 168

What is the error in the following theophylline case study? An asthmatic patient was taking theophylline three times a day. A plasma level measurement three hours after one particular morning dose indicated 15 μg/ml of theophylline. Unfortunately, the patient reported breathing probems occurring frequently in the last two hours before afternoon or evening doses were due. The doctor recommended

1. increasing the dose by 50% in the hope of stopping the breathing difficulties
2. that sustained-release theophylline was too expensive
3. taking theophylline four times a day, as an alternative to (1)
4. the use of an electronic device to check the patient's compliance

Answer   ⓔ

Answer 1 is incorrect because it would have led to peaks above 20 μg/ml and an excessive risk of drug toxicity. Answer 2 is incorrect, because sustained-release theophylline is an excellent way of damping-down fluctuation between peaks and troughs—it is possible to extend the dosing interval to 12 hours or even more with such preparations. Taking theophylline four times a day is just not practicable (answer 3). Answer 4 is a good idea, if expensive fun, but since the patient only experienced breathing difficulties in the later part of any dosing interval, it is doubtful whether compliance was a problem. Thus all four statements are true, in that they contributed to the error.

PROBLEM 169

What are the errors/problems in the following case study? A 29-year-old mother of two children was using oral contraceptives and experienced a single isolated seizure, following which she was prescribed phenytoin. One year later she became pregnant. The phenytoin concentration in plasma at the time was 5.4 μg/ml, and

her doctor immediately doubled her phenytoin dose, to raise her
level above the threshold of 10 μg/ml.

1. The phenytoin neutralized the oral contraceptive effect by
   enzyme induction.
2. The oral contraceptives caused low phenytoin levels, by
   enzyme induction.
3. The patient should not have had her phenytoin dose
   doubled, as this would almost certainly more than double
   the plasma concentration because of nonlinear pharmacokinetics
4. The patient should not have had her phenytoin dose
   doubled, because pregnant women should receive the
   lowest phenytoin dose possible consistent with seizure
   control, regardless of levels.

Answer $\boxed{e}$

This is a chapter of accidents resulting from ignorance. All four
errors/problems probably occurred. The only doubt would be
whether the low phenytoin levels were caused by the oral contraceptives. Some authorities would even say that no patient should
receive phenytoin for a long period after just one seizure.

PROBLEM 170

The following are good reasons for monitoring phenytoin.

1. Narrow therapeutic range
2. Plasma levels correlate with effect and toxicity
3. There is wide interpatient variation in kinetics
4. Absorption is non-linear

Answer $\boxed{a}$

Phenytoin dose have a narrow therapeutic range, plasma levels do
correlate well with toxicity, and there is a wide interpatient variation in kinetics. Metabolism, not absorption is non-linear, so that 1,
2, and 3 are correct.

PROBLEM 171

Which of the following assumptions are made when using a *single point* method of dosing phenytoin?

1. that the population Km applies in the patient in question
2. that the population V_{max} applies in the patient in question
3. that Michaelis–Menten kinetics apply
4. that the relation between Km and dose is linear.

Answer ⓑ

Single point approaches make the assumption that Michaelis–Menten kinetics apply and that the population Km can be used. The population V_{max} is not used, and in no sense is there a linear relation between Km and dose. Thus 1 and 3 are correct.

PROBLEM 172

Hydrochlorothiazine is believed to have saturable absorption processes. As the result of this:

1. increasing the dose will lead to a disproportionately large increase in plasma concentrations
2. lower doses will be absorbed at faster rates than higher doses
3. higher doses will have higher rate constants of metabolism
4. higher doses will have an increased chance of being partially excreted in feces

Answer ⓓ

Answer 1 is not correct, as increasing the dose will lead to disproportionately *small* increases in plasma concentrations. Lower doses will not be absorbed faster; when a process tends towards saturation, it still shows an increased rate of occurrence. Answer 3 refers to metabolism, not absorption. Answer 4 is correct; as the dose increases, lesser proportions of higher doses are absorbed. All the residues can do is be excreted.

PART V:
Questions Relating to Specific Scientific Papers

In this part of the book use the code on page 133.

PROBLEM 173

In their paper on the influence of age on theophylline clearance, Randolph *et al.* (1986)

1. reported that there is conflict in the literature concerning the effect of age on theophylline kinetics
2. studied thirty healthy male volunteers in three age groups
3. showed that clearance measurements were significantly correlated with age
4. showed that age alone accounted for only 31% of the variability in clearance

Answer   [e]

All four statements are correct.

Reference

Randolph, V.C., Seaman, J.J., Dickson, B., Peace, K.E., Frand, W.O., and Young, M.D. The effect of age on theophylline clearance in normal subjects. *Br. J. Clin. Pharmacol. 22*, 603–605 (1986).

PROBLEM 174

In their paper on imipramine demethylation and hydroxylation in relation to sparteine oxidation phenotype, Brosen *et al.* (1986) showed that

1. 2-hydroxylation of imipramine and desipramine is dependent mainly on the sparteine oxygenase
2. demethylation is dependent mainly on an isozyme different from that responsible for hydroxylation
3. a sparteine phenotype test would be useful in selecting initial doses in imipramine therapy
4. their results could be extrapolated to other antidepressants including amitriptyline

Answer   [a]

Statements 1, 2, and 3 are correct.

Reference

Brosen, K., Otton, S.V., and Gram, L.F. Imipramine demethylation and hydroxylation: impact of the sparteine oxidation phenotype. *Clin. Pharmacol. Ther.* 40, 544–549 (1986).

PROBLEM 175

The scientific literature concerning links between obesity and pharmacokinetics leads to the following conclusions:

1. there is little or no evidence supporting belief in a general increase or reduction in activity of drug metabolic or excretory processes in obese patients
2. adjustments in doses related to actual weight are likely to be to loading doses only
3. maintenance dose adjustment should relate to ideal body weight (IBW)
4. In the equation, dosing weight (DW) = IBW + xEBW (where EBW is excess body weight), x is 1 for low volume of distribution drugs such as benzodiazepines

Answer ⓔ

All four statements are correct.

References

Krishnaswamy, K., and Sri, U. The effect of malnutrition on the pharmacokinetics of phenylbutazone. *Clin. Pharmacokinetics* 6, 152–159 (1981).

Krishnaswamy, K. In *Handbook of Clinical Pharmacokinetics* (Gibaldi, M., and Prescott, L., eds.). New York: Adis Press, 1983, Section II, pp. 216–242.

Benedek, I.H., Fiske, W.D., Griffin, W.O., Bell, R.M., Blouin, R.A., and McNamara, P.J. Serum α_1-acid glycoprotein and the binding of drugs in obesity. *Br. J. Clin. Pharmacol.* 16, 751–754 (1984).

Bauer, L.A., Wareing-Tran, C., Edwards, W.A.D., Raisys, V., Ferreri, L., Jack, R., Dellinger, E.P., and Simonowitz, D. Cimetidine clearance in the obese. *Clin. Pharmacol. Ther.* 37, 425–430 (1985).

PROBLEM 176

In their paper on lidocaine disposition in men and women, Wing *et al.* reported that

1. the lidocaine half-life was longer in women
2. there was no protein binding difference
3. Vd_{ss} was lower in men
4. systematic clearance was the same in both men and women

Answer [e]

All four statements are correct.

References

Wing, L.M.H., Miners, J.O., Birkett, D.J., Foenander, T., Lillywhite, K., and Wanwinolcuk, S. Lidocaine disposition—sex differences and effects of cimetidine. *Clin. Pharmacol. Ther. 35,* 695–701 (1984).
Richardson, C.J., Blocka, K.L.N., Ross, S.G., and Verbeeck, R.K. Effects of age and sex on piroxicam disposition. *Clin. Pharmacol. Ther. 37,* 13–18 (1985).

PROBLEM 177

Which of the following statements are true in relation to physical fitness exercise and posture effects on pharmacokinetics?

1. Training for athletic activity leads to relatively fast antipyrine metabolism.
2. Exercise causes a relatively rapid release of drugs from intramuscular depot injection sites.
3. There is a decrease in estimated hepatic blood flow (EHBF) on changing from the supine to the upright position.
4. Nitroglycerin plasma levels are relatively high when recorded in the supine as opposed to the standing position.

Answer [e]

All four statements are correct.

References

Boel, J., Andersen, L.B., Rasmussen, B., Hansen, S.H., and Døssing, M. Hepatic drug metabolism and physical fitness. *Clin. Pharmacol. Ther.* 36, 121–126 (1984).
Curry, S.H., and Kwon, H.R. Influence of posture on plasma nitroglycerin. *Br. J. Clin. Pharmacol.* 19, 403–404 (1985).

PROBLEM 178

In the literature concerned with effects of pregnancy on pharmacokinetic properties of drugs, it is reported that:

1. the rate of metabolism of phenytoin is relatively high in pregnancy
2. the renal elimination rate of lithium is relatively high in pregnancy
3. renal blood flow, GFR, and Cl_{cr} increase, at least in early pregnancy
4. unusually high levels of digoxin occur in pregnancy

Answer [a]

Statements 1, 2, and 3 are correct.

References

Yoshikawa, T., Sugiyama, Y., Sawada, Y., Iga, T., Hanaro, M., Kawasaki, S., and Yanagida, M. Effect of late pregnancy on salicylate, diazepam, warfarin and propranolol binding: use of fluorescent probes. *Clin. Pharmacol. Ther.* 36, 201–208 (1984).
Hogstedt, S., Lindberg, B., Peng, D.R., Regårdh, C-G., and Rane, A. Pregnancy-induced increase in metoprolol metabolism. *Clin. Pharmacol. Ther.* 37, 688–692 (1985).
Foulds, G., Miller, D., Knirsch, A.K., and Thrupp. L.D. Sulbactam kinetics and excretion into breast milk in postpartum women. *Clin. Pharmacol. Ther.* 38, 692–696 (1985).

PROBLEM 179

In liver disease

1. azotemia leads to reduced binding of thiopentone to plasma protein
2. hypergammaglobulinemia leads to increased binding of d-tubocurarine
3. hepatotoxicity of acetaminophen is increased in patients treated with enzyme-inducing agents beforehand
4. enzyme induction is a greater influence on the kinetics of phenylbutazone than is the liver problem itself

Answer ⸤e⸥

All four statements are correct.

References

Meredith, C.G., Christian, C.D., Johnson, R.F., Madhaven, S.V., and Schenker, S. Diphenhydramine disposition in chronic liver disease. *Clin. Pharmacol. Ther. 35*, 474–479 (1984).
Blaschke, T.F., In *Handbook of Clinical Pharmacokinetics* (Gibaldi, M., and Prescott, L., eds.). New York: Adis Press, 1983, Section III, pp. 126–139.
Maxwell, J.D., Carrella, M., Parkes, J.D., Williams, R., Mould, G.P., and Curry, S.H. Plasma disappearance and cerebral effects of chlorpramazine in cirrhosis. *Clin. Sci. 43*, 143–151 (1972).

PROBLEM 180

The following are approximately correct, clinically desirable ranges for the drugs mentioned under the conditions described:

1. phenytoin (dilantin), 10–20 μg/ml, based on sampling at uncontrolled times
2. procaine amide, 5–10 μg/ml, based on sampling at uncontrolled times

3. lithium, 0.8–1.5 mmol/liter, based on the minimum concentration during the fluctuating steady state or 12 hours post-dosage

4. digoxin, 0.52–2 μg/ml, based on sampling at uncontrolled times

Answer [a]

Statements 1, 2, and 3 are correct.

References

Evans, W.E., Shentag, J.J., and Jusko, W.J. (eds.), *Applied Pharmacokinetics*. San Francisco: Applied Therapeutics, Inc., 1980.

Winter, M.E. *Basic Clinical Pharmacokinetics*. San Francisco: Applied Therapeutics, Inc., 1980.

Curry, S.H. Drug assay in therapeutic monitoring, *Trends in Analytical Chemistry 5*, 102–105 (1986).

PROBLEM 181

Gentamicin monitoring involves or has as its objective

1. measurement of the gentamicin half-life in the second of the two or three phases of plasma level decline seen after i.v. doses

2. peak concentrations of approximately 8 μg/ml, measured not earlier than 1 h after i.m. doses

3. trough concentrations below 2 μg/ml

4. prevention of oto- and nephrotoxicity

Answer [e]

All four statements are correct.

References

Yee, G.C., and Evans, W.E. Reappraisal of guidelines for pharmacokinetic monitoring of aminoglycosides. *Pharmacotherapy 1*, 55–75 (1981).

Curry, S.H. Drug assay in therapeutic monitoring. *Trends in Analytical Chemistry 5*, 102–105 (1986).

PROBLEM 182

In the literature concerned with effects of thyroid disease on drug response, it is reported that

1. antipyrine metabolism is accelerated in the hyperthyroid state
2. there is an unexpected slowing of phenytoin metabolism in the hyperthyroid state
3. it may be necessary to increase warfarin doses in hypothyroids because of metabolite handling of vitamin K-dependent clotting factor
4. the systematic clearance (Cl_s) of propranolol is greater in patients with thyrotoxicosis compared with euthyroid patients

Answer   e

All four statements are correct.

References

Wells, P.G., Feely, J., Wilkinson, G.R., and Wood, A.J.J. Effect of thyrotoxicosis on liver blood flow and propranolol disposition after long-term dosing. *Clin. Pharmacol. Ther. 33*, 603–608 (1983).
Eichelbaum, M. Drug metabolism in thyroid disease, in *Handbook of Clinical Pharmacokinetics* (Gibaldi, M., and Prescott, L., eds.). New York: Adis Press, 1983, Section III, pp. 169–181.

PROBLEM 183

The following physiological factors cause the pharmacological effects listed:

1. reduced gastric acid secretion in persons over 65 years of age—increased absorption of acidic drugs

2. undeveloped renal tubular transport mechanism at birth—prolonged retention of penicillin in the body
3. excessive skin permeability in young children—brain effects caused by bathing in hexachlorophene
4. a combination of changes in liver activity and CNS sensitivity—exceptional CNS depression in elderly people treated with benzodiazepines

Answer [e]

All four statements are correct.

References

Crooks, J., and Stevenson, I.H. *Drugs and the Elderly*. London: Macmillan, 1979.
Morselli, P.L., Franco-Morselli, R., and Bassi, L. Clinical pharmacokinetics in newborns and infants. Age-related differences and therapeutic implication. *Clin. Pharmacokinetics, 5*, 485–527 (1980).
Greenblatt, D.J., Allen, M.D., Harmatz, J.S., and Shader, R.I. Diazepam disposition determinants. *Clin. Pharmacol. Ther. 27*, 301–312 (1980).

PROBLEM 184

The literature on drug disposition in the neonate indicates that

1. renal excretion of penicillin is slower at birth than 30 days later
2. phenytoin metabolism is slower at birth compared with later
3. theophylline is metabolized to caffeine more rapidly in neonates than in adults
4. digoxin binding to plasma proteins is less than in adults

Answer [e]

All four statements are correct.

References

Rajchot, P. Toward optimization of therapy in the neonate. *Clin. Pharmacol. Ther. 33*, 551–555 (1984).
Morselli, P.L. In *Handbook of Clinical Pharmacokinetics* (Gibaldi, M., and Prescott, L., eds.). New York: Adis Press, 1983, Section III, pp. 79–97.

PROBLEM 185

Which of the following statements are true?

1. Congestive heart failure causes relatively fast metabolism of lidocaine.
2. Myocardial infarction causes an increase in binding of disopyramide to plasma protein.
3. Heparin injection (i.v.) causes decreased plasma free fatty acid concentrations and therefore increased binding of propranolol to plasma proteins.
4. Achlorhydria results in impaired (either slower or lower overall total) absorption of aspirin.

Answer   ⊡

Statements 2 and 4 are correct.

References

Paxton, J.W., and Norris, R.M. Propranolol disposition after acute myocardial infarction. *Clin. Pharmacol. Ther. 36* 337–342 (1984).
Williams L., and Benet, L.Z. Drug pharmacokinetics in cardiac and hepatic diseases. *Ann. Rev. Pharmacol. Toxicol. 20*, 389–413 (1980).
Parsons, R.L. In *Handbook of Clinical Pharmacokinetics* (Gibaldi, M., and Prescott, L., eds.). New York: Adis Press, 1983, Section III, pp. 17–33.

PROBLEM 186

Which of the following statements are true?

1. Tetracycline absorption is reduced by milk.
2. Digoxin absorption is slowed by food.
3. Theophylline concentrations in blood are reduced by consumption of charcoal-broiled beef because of an increased rate of metabolism.
4. Griseofulvin absorption occurs more rapidly if the dose accompanies a fatty meal.

Answer ⒠

All four are correct.

References

Karim, A., Burns, T., Wearley, L., Streicher, J., and Palmer, M. Food-induced changes in theophylline absorption from controlled-release formulations. *Clin. Pharmacol. Ther. 38*, 77–83 (1985).
Toothaker, R.D., and Welling, P.G. The effect of food on drug bioavailability. *Ann. Rev. Pharmacol. Toxicol. 20*, 173–199 (1980).

PROBLEM 187

Which of the following statements are true?

1. In laboratory animals, sugar intake decreases P-450 activity and prolongs hexobarbital sleeping times.
2. In laboratory animals, a shortage of protein decreases P-450 activity.
3. In humans, a low carbohydrate/high protein diet reduces the half-life of antipyrine.
4. In humans, malnutrition decreases plasma albumin and decreases the half-life of phenylbutazone.

Answer ⒠

All four statements are correct.

References

Krishnaswamy, I., and Sri, U. The effect of malnutrition on the pharmacokinetics of phenylbutazone. *Clin. Pharmacokinetics 6*, 152–159 (1981).

Krishnaswamy, K. In *Handbook of Clinical Pharmacokinetics* (Gibaldi, M., and Prescott, L., eds.). New York: Adis Press, 1983, Section II, pp. 216–242.

PROBLEM 188

Which of the following statements are true?

1. Theophylline trough levels are generally higher in the morning than in the evening (when patients are treated with doses every 12 hours).
2. The valproate free fraction is relatively high during the night because of competition with fatty acids for binding sites on plasma proteins.
3. The urinary pH is relatively low in the morning (provided the person concerned did not eat a late night meal) and this leads to relatively fast renal excretion of meperidine administered in the morning.
4. Debrisoquine can be used to assess the activity of microsomal drug metabolizing enzymes, from the ratio of debrisoquine to 4-hydroxydebrisoquine concentrations in a carefully timed urine sample following a test dose.

Answer ⓔ

All four statements are correct.

References

Bauer, L.A., Davis, R., Wilensky, A., Raisys, V., and Levy, R.H. Diurnal variation in valproic acid clearance. *Clin. Pharmacol. Ther. 35*, 505–509 (1984).

Editorial. Polymorphic drug oxidation—much ado about nothing? *Lancet ii*, p. 1337, (June 16, 1984).

St-Pierre, M.V., Spino, M., Isles, A.F., Tesoro, A., and MacLeod, S.M. Temporal variation in the disposition of theophylline and its metabolites. *Clin. Pharmacol. Ther. 38*, 89–95 (1985).

PROBLEM 189

Which of the following statements are true?

1. Gastroenteritis in children can cause acidosis and a decrease in urinary pH leading to a decreased rate of renal elimination of sulfonamides.
2. Hypothyroidism causes vasodilation, plus an increase in heart rate, leading to an increase in tissue perfusion and slower metabolism of propranolol.
3. Halothane but not enflurane is metabolized relatively slowly in hypothyroid rats.
4. Riboflavin shows especially slow urinary excretion in hypothroid children when given by intramuscular injection.

Answer b

Statements 2 and 4 are correct.

References

Wells, P.G., Feely, J., Wilkinson, G.R., and Wood, A.J.J. The effect of thyrotoxicosis on liver blood flow and propranolol disposition after long-term dosing. *Clin. Pharmacol. Ther. 33*, 603–608 (1983).
Nimmo, W.S. In *Handbook of Clinical Pharmacokinetics* (Gibaldi, M., and Prescott, L., eds.). New York: Adis Press, 1983, Section III, pp. 1–16.
Parsons, R.L. In *Handbook of Clinical Pharmacokinetics* (Gibaldi, M., and Prescott, L., eds.). New York: Adis Press, 1983, Section III, pp. 17–33.

PROBLEM 190

Which of the following statements are true?

1. Phenylbutazone is metabolized relatively rapidly by patients with cirrhosis because of enzyme induction.
2. Tolbutamide is metabolized relatively rapidly in acute

      viral hepatitis because of reduced binding to plasma protein.

3. Chlorpromazine causes especially dramatic effects in patients with liver disorders primarily because of end-organ sensitivity.

4. Succinylcholine causes especially long apnea in patients with liver disorders.

Answer   [e]

All four statements are correct.

References

Meredith, C.G., Christian, C.D., Johnson, R.F., Madhaven, S.V., and Schenker, S. Diphenhydramine disposition in chronic liver disease. *Clin. Pharmacol. Ther.* 35, 474–479 (1984).

Blaschke, T.F. In *Handbook of Clinical Pharmacokinetics* (Gibaldi, M., and Prescott, L., eds.). New York: Adis Press, 1983, Section III, pp. 126–139.

Maxwell, J.D., Carrella, M., Parkes, J.D., Williams, R., Mould, G.P., and Curry, S.H. Plasma disappearance and cerebral effects of chlorpromazine in cirrhosis. *Clin. Sci.* 43, 143–151 (1972).

PROBLEM 191

Which of the following statements are true?

1. Benzodiazepines should be administered in low doses to old people primarily because of end-organ sensitivity factors.

2. The effect of succinylcholine correlates closely with its hydrolysis rate by plasma pseudocholinesterases.

3. The activity of the enzymes responsible for the metabolism of succinylcholine can be evaluated using the dibucaine number concept.

4. The half-life of ampicillin becomes gradually greater as children pass from less than 2 days to more than 65 days old.

Answer   [a]

Statements 1, 2, and 3 are correct.

References

Rajchot, P. Toward optimization of therapy in the neonate. *Clin. Pharmacol. Ther.* 33, 551–555 (1984).

Luderer, J.R., Patel, I.H., Durkin, J., and Schneck, D.W. Age and cetmoxane kinetics. *Clin. Pharmacol. Ther.* 35, 19–25 (1984).

Schaad, U.B., Hayton, W.L., and Stoeckel, K. Single-dose cefriaxone kinetics in the new-born. *Clin. Pharmacol. Ther.* 37, 522–528 (1985).

PROBLEM 192

In a drug analysis

1. precision refers to scatter about a mean
2. accuracy refers to the closeness of an estimated mean to the real value
3. specificity refers to the need for the analysis to be of a single defined compound
4. blank refers to the signal in the detection system arising when no drug is present

Answer [e]

All four statements are correct.

References

Smith, R.V. Determination of drugs and metabolites in biological fluids. *Trends in Analytical Chemistry 3*, 178–181 (1984).

Curry, S.H. Drug assay in therapeutic monitoring. *Trends in Analytical Chemistry 5*, 102–105 (1986).

PROBLEM 193

Which of the following statements are true?

1. The process of pharmacokinetic iterative computing invol-

ves repeated testing of estimates of possible pharmacokinetic parameters against real data in the search for
the best fit.

2. Simulation involves generation of predicted data points
from defined parameter values.

3. Data analysis involves the use of defined points in the
search for reliable estimates of parameter values.

4. Iteration is a feature of the NLIN, NONLIN, and PCNON-
LIN programs.

Answer ⒠

All four statements are correct.

References

Barlow, R.B. *Biodata Handling with Microcomputers*. Cambridge:
Elsevier Biosoft, 1983.

Curry, S.H., and Thakker, K.M. Pharmacokinetic simulations with
hand-held programmable calculators. *Trends in Pharmacological Sci-
ences 6*, 122–123 (1985).

Curry, S.H., Laizure, C.S., and DeVare, C.L. Spread-sheet analysis in
pharmacokinetic simulations. *Trends in Pharmacological Scineces 7*,
220–223 (1986).

Metzler, C.M., and Weiner, D.L. A User's Manual for NONLIN and
Associated Programs. The Upjohn Co., Kalamazoo, Michigan, 1984.

SAS User's Guide Version 5 Edition, SAS Institute, Raleigh, North
Carolina, 1985.

Appendix

References and Further Reading

1. Albert, K.S., (ed.). *Drug Absorption and Disposition: Statistical Considerations.* Washington D.C.: American Pharmaceutical Association, 1980.
2. Benet, L.Z., Massoud, N., and Gambertoglio, J.G. *Pharmacokinetic Basis for Drug Treatment.* New York: Raven Press, 1983.
3. Brodie, B.B. Physicochemical and biochemical aspects of pharmacology. *J. Am. Med. Assoc. 13,* 660–663 (1967).
4. Curry, S.H. *Drug Disposition and Pharmacokinetics,* 3rd ed. Oxford: Blackwell; St. Louis: Mosby, 1980.
5. Curry, S.H., and Whelpton, R.W. *Manual of Laboratory Pharmacokinetics.* New York: Wiley, 1983.
6. Dost, F.H. Der Blutspiegel—Kinetic der Konzentrationsablaufe in der Drieslaffussigkeit. Leipzig: G. Thieme, 1953.
7. Evans, W.E., Shentag, J.J., and Jusko, W.J. (eds.). *Applied Pharmacokinetics: Principles of Therapeutic Drug Monitoring.* San Francisco: Applied Therapeutics, Inc., (3rd. ed., 1986).
8. Gibaldi, M. *Biopharmaceutics and Clinical Pharmacokinetics,* 3rd ed. Philadelphia: Lea and Febiger, 1983.
9. Gibaldi, M., and Perrier, D. *Pharmacokinetics,* New York: Marcel Dekker, 1975. [2nd ed., 1982.]
10. Holford, N.H.G., and Sheiner, L.B. Kinetics of pharmacologic response, *Pharmacol. Ther. 16,* 143–166 (1982).
11. Kruger-Thiemer, E. Dosage schedules and pharmacokinetics in chemotherapy. *J. Am. Pharm. Assoc. (Sci. Ed.) 49,* 311–313 (1960).
12. LaDu, B.N., Mandel, H.G., and Way, E.L. *Fundamentals of Drug Metabolism and Drug Disposition,* Baltimore: Williams and Wilkins, 1971.
13. Levy, G. Kinetics of pharmacologic effects. *Clin. Pharmacol. Ther. 7,* 362–372 (1966).
14. Mungal, D.R. *Applied Clinical Pharmacokinetics.* New York: Raven Press, 1983.
15. Nelson, E. Kinetics of drug absorption, distribution, metabolism and excretion. *J. Pharm. Sci. 50,* 181–192 (1961).
16. Niazi, S. *Textbook of Biopharmaceutics and Clinical Pharmacokinetics.* New York: Appleton-Century-Crofts, 1979.
17. Notari, R.E. *Biopharmaceutics and Pharmacokinetics: An Introduction,* 3rd ed. New York, Marcel Dekker, 1982.
18. Ritschel, W.A. *Graphic Approach to Clinical Pharmacokinetics.* New York: J.R. Prous, 1983.
19. Rowland, M., and Tozer, T. *Clinical Pharmacokinetics.* Philadelphia: Lea and Febiger, 1980.
20. Rowland, M., and Tucker, G. Symbols in pharmacokinetics. *J. Pharmacokinetics Biopharmaceutics 8,* 497–507 (1980).
21. Shargel, L., and Yu, A.B.C. *Applied Biopharmaceutics and Pharmacokinetics.* New York: Appleton-Century-Crofts, 1980. [2nd ed., 1985.]
22. Teorell, T. Kinetics of distribution of substances administered to the body I. The extravascular modes of administration. *Arch. Int. Pharmacodyn. Ther. 57,* 205–225 (1937).

181

23. Teorell, T. Kinetics of distribution of substances administered to the body II. The intravascular modes of administration. *Arch. Int. Pharmacodyn. Ther. 57*, 226–240 (1937).

24. Wagner, J.G. *Biopharmaceutics and Relevant Pharmacokinetics.* Hamilton, Illinois: Drug Intelligence Publications (Hamilton), 1971.

25. Wagner, J.G. *Fundamentals of Clinical Pharmacokinetics*, Hamilton, Illinois: Drug Intelligence Publications (Hamilton), 1975.

26. Wagner, J.G. History of pharmacokinetics, *Pharmacol. Ther. 12*, 537–562 (1981).

27. Winter, M.E. *Basic Clinical Pharmacokinetics.* San Francisco: Applied Therapeutics, Inc., 1980.

28. Wilkinson, G.R., and Shand, D.G. Commentary: a physiological approach to drug clearance. *Clin. Pharmacol. Ther. 18*, 377–390 (1975).

INDEX